The Lost
HERBAL REMEDY

For Beginners

Nature's Pharmacy: A Comprehensive Handbook to Effective Herbal
Remedies for Common Ailments

Perry C. Buck

CONTENTS

Chapter 6

Chapter 7

Chapter 8

Chapter 1
Introduction

In the forgotten corners of the world, amidst ancient scrolls and whispered legends, lies a secret known to few—the ancient art of herbal remedies. "The Lost Book of The Herbal Remedy for Beginners" is your gateway to this mystical world, a treasure trove of knowledge that has been passed down through generations, yet remains largely untouched by the modern hand. This book is not just a guide; it's an invitation to embark on a journey of discovery, to reconnect with the wisdom of our ancestors, and to harness the healing power of nature.

As you turn these pages, you will be introduced to the hidden language of plants and herbs, learning how to listen and respond to the subtle cues of the natural world. From the humble dandelion to the majestic oak, every plant has a story to tell and a remedy to offer. You will discover how to prepare potions, salves, and teas that heal and rejuvenate, using ingredients that are often found not in the far reaches of some exotic land, but in your own backyard.

"The Lost Book of The Herbal Remedy for Beginners" demystifies the ancient practices and makes them accessible to the modern seeker. It offers a gentle, yet profound introduction to the art of herbal healing, emphasizing the importance of living in harmony with nature. Whether you are a novice eager to explore the healing properties of herbs or a seasoned practitioner seeking to deepen your knowledge, this book will serve as a faithful guide on your journey.

Embark on this enchanting voyage into the heart of herbalism, where each page turned is a step closer to unlocking the secrets of the earth. Welcome to the beginning of your transformative journey with "The Lost Book of The Herbal Remedy for Beginners."

"Herbal" refers to a product made from plants, while "medicine" refers to something that can harmonize, heal, or prevent disease. So, "herbal medicine" refers to chemicals derived from plants that can be used to treat, prevent, or provide nutrition. Ayurveda and herbal medicine work together in this branch, which includes all areas of herbal medicine that have to do with plants, pharmacognosy, phytochemistry, phytotherapy, botanical medicines, Ayurveda, natural chemistry, agriculture science, Unani medicine, biotechnology, and biochemistry. Someone who works with plants, especially herbs used for medicine, is called a herbalist. Herbal journals write about how plants can be used to treat illness.

It is possible to use plants as medicine. Herbal medicines help people stay healthy or get better when they are sick. People use them to ease their complaints, get more energy, unwind, or lose weight.

Herbal medicines are not tested or controlled like medicines are.

What do you know about what you're getting and whether it's useful? This guide can help you pick out safe herbs and use them.

Herbs aren't medicines.

When you use a herbal medicine, you need to be careful. Herbal medicines are a type of food supplement. They're not medicines. What you need to know about herbals is this:

- Because they are not medicines, herbs are not controlled.
- Herbs don't have to be checked in a strict way before they can be sold.
- Herbs might not work the way they're said to.
- No one has to give their approval for labels
- The label might not have the right amount of an ingredient. Some herbal remedies might have extra ingredients or contaminants that aren't mentioned.

How to Pick Safe Herbal Medicines and Use Them

Herbs can help you stay fit and feel better. But you need to understand how to buy things. When picking plant medicines, use these tips.

- Pay close attention to what the product says to do. How would you describe the product? Does the pill really "melt away" fat? Do you think it will work faster than normal care? Do your doctor and drug makers not want you to know this secret? These kinds of claims are red flags. It's likely not true if something sounds too good to be true.
- Keep in mind that "true stories" are not proof of anything science. A lot of goods use real-life stories to get people to buy them. Some people might get the same quote, but that doesn't mean that other people will too.

- Talk to your provider about a product before you try it. Ask them what they think. Is it safe to use? How likely is it that it will work? Are there risks? Does it work with other medicines? Will it get in the way of your treatment?

- Only buy from companies that have tags that say things like "USP Verified" or "ConsumerLab.com Approved Quality." Companies that have these licenses agree to test their products to make sure they are pure and of good quality.

- If you are over 65, don't give herbal pills to kids or use them yourself. First, talk to your service provider.

- If you are taking medicine, don't use herbs until you talk to your doctor.

- Don't use them if you are pregnant or nursing.

- Don't use them before or after surgery.

- Tell your doctor or nurse every time you take herbals. They might change the way your drugs work or the care you get.

Chapter 2

What Is Herbal Medicine?

Natural chemicals found in plants that are used to treat illness as part of local or regional healing practices are called herbal medicines. These items are complicated mixes of natural chemicals that can come from any part of a plant, whether it is raw or prepared.

All over the world, people have used herbs for healing for a very long time. There are many types of traditional medicine, and their beliefs and methods are affected by society, the environment, and where they are located. However, they all agree on one thing: life should be looked at as a whole. Traditional Chinese Medicine and Ayurvedic Medicine are two well-known types of plant medicine. They are based on the idea that health should be valued more than illness. People can get better and focus on their general health when they use healing herbs instead of just one illness that usually happens when the mind, body, and environment are out of balance.

In homeopathy and botanical medicine, people have used plants for thousands of years, and they are still useful in the current Western world. The World Health Organization recently said that herbal medicines are used by about 80% of people around the world as part of their primary health care. The yearly market for these products is close to $60 billion. In the US, people are interested in herbal treatment more because the cost of prescription drugs is going up and people are interested in natural or organic remedies again.

Herbs that are whole have a lot of ingredients that are used to treat illnesses and ease their effects. Herbal medicine, which is also known as herbal medicine, uses the seeds, berries, roots, leaves, bark, or flowers of a plant to treat illness. The biological features of these plants are good for you. Other things, like the type of setting the plant grew in, how it was harvested, and how it was processed, are also to blame for their benefits. The plant is sold either whole or as an extract, which means that some of the chemicals have been taken out by mashing it with water, alcohol, or other solvents. Dozens of chemicals are found in the end products, such as sterols, alkaloids, flavonoids, glycosides, saponins, and fatty acids.

Benefits of Herbal Medicine

1. Not as expensive as regular medicine

Some things in modern medicine are very expensive, and medicines are no different. People simply can't afford to pay for their medicine every month, which is one reason why plant medicine is becoming more popular.

A study in the journal Evidence-Based Complementary and Alternative Medicine looked at whether natural health items are a good way to treat illness that doesn't cost too much. Researchers discovered that natural health products may save people money when compared to surgery and other problems that can happen afterward. More study is needed to find out if herbal products are more cost-effective than pharmaceuticals in other areas of modern medicine, but early data suggests that this is the case.

2. It's easier to get than prescription drugs.

You don't need a prescription to buy herbal products like herbal teas, essential oils, and herbal extracts. You can find them in most health food stores and even some grocery shops. This makes it easy to get herbal products and keeps you from having to pay more for health care.

Herbs are dietary supplements, which means they don't need to be approved by the FDA before they are made, sold, or promoted. It's up to us as consumers to choose between the competitors, even though this makes it easier to buy and use these useful goods. Before taking any herbal product, make sure you read the labels and ingredients very carefully. Buy from a company with a good reputation that guarantees the product is 100% pure-grade.

3.   Have healing and helpful properties

Herbs are used to treat both long-term and short-term illnesses and conditions, including major health problems like heart disease, prostate issues, sadness, inflammation, and a weak immune system. Herbs are used to treat illnesses and situations all over the world, and many studies have shown that they work. More than 70% of the 177 drugs allowed around the world to treat cancer are based on natural products or chemicals that look like natural products.

Top Herbs Used in Herbal Medicine

1. Raw Garlic

Flavonoids, oligosaccharides, selenium, allicin, and high amounts of sulfur are just some of the important nutrients that garlic has. Whether you eat it raw or cooked, garlic can help treat diabetes, reduce inflammation, boost your immune system, keep your blood pressure in check, protect against heart disease, ease allergy symptoms, fight fungal and viral infections, and stop hair loss.

Cardiovascular disease is the top cause of death in the United States. Studies show that eating garlic makes cardiovascular disease worse. According to a study in the Journal of Nutrition, garlic lowers cholesterol, stops platelets from sticking together, lowers blood pressure, and boosts antioxidant levels.

2. Ginger

Ginger is the most popular food seasoning in the world right now. Gingerols, an oily fluid from the root that works as a powerful antioxidant and anti-inflammatory, are what give ginger its health benefits. Ginger has many bioactive compounds that can help with digestion and nausea, as well as the immune system and lungs. They can also fight bacterial and fungal infections, treat stomach ulcers, ease pain, improve diabetes, stop malabsorption, and maybe even stop the growth of cancer cells.

According to a 2013 review of the evidence published in the International Journal of Preventive Medicine, ginger has a lot of proof that it can help fight cancer. Its active ingredients, such as gingerols, shogaol, and paradols, are what can help prevent different types of cancer. Researchers also found that ginger can slow down the aging process by reducing inflammation and protecting cells from damage.

Ginger can be used in many ways. If you want to eat it raw, you can take it as a vitamin or powder, make a tea with it, or put oil on your skin.

3. Turmeric

Turmeric comes from a plant that has been used as medicine for almost 4,000 years. Over 3,000 articles about turmeric show that modern medicine has started to understand how important it is. You can add this strong plant to any recipe or take it by itself. Turmeric has many health benefits, such as the ability to stop or slow blood clotting, fight sadness, lower inflammation, ease the pain of arthritis, control diabetes, treat digestive problems, lower cholesterol, and fight cancer.

Several studies have shown that turmeric is a powerful antioxidant, anti-inflammatory, antimutagenic, antibacterial, and anticancer substance. Turmeric products are antioxidants that can get rid of free radicals, boost antioxidant enzymes, and stop lipid peroxidation.

4. Ginger and ginseng

Ginseng is one of the most well-known plant medicines in the world. It has been used for hundreds of years in both Asia and North America. Native Americans used the root as a stimulant and to treat headaches. They also used it to treat infertility, fever, and stomach problems.

The Brain Performance and Nutrition Research Centre in the UK did the study. was done to find out more about ginseng's benefits and how it can help with mental health and happiness. Thirty volunteers took 200 milligrams of ginseng and a placebo three times each. The data showed that taking ginseng for eight days not only slowed down the mood drop but also made it harder for the volunteers to do mental math. During the eight-day treatment, the 400-milligram amount made people feel calmer and helped them do math better.

People also use ginseng to lower their blood sugar, treat sexual problems, treat stress, help them lose weight, improve lung function, boost their immune systems, and lower inflammation. Ginseng can be bought as a tea, a powder, a pill, or a tablet.

5. Milk Thistle

Herbal medicines made from milk thistle products have been used for almost 2,000 years. There are a lot of lipophilic products from the seeds of the milk thistle plant. These are bioflavonoids that boost the immune system and slow down oxidative stress. In addition, the plant is used to treat inflammation. It can help the digestive system work better, make more bile, improve skin health, slow down the aging process, lower cholesterol, and clean out the body.

A study that looked at the safety and effectiveness of milk thistle found that it can help protect against some types of cancer. The plant can also be used to help people with liver diseases, hepatitis C, HIV, diabetes, and high cholesterol. It is also known that milk thistle extracts, which are often sold in pill form, are safe and well-tolerated.

6. A feverfew

Fetifew has been used for hundreds of years to treat fevers, headaches, stomachaches, toothaches, bug bites, impotence, and problems with periods and labor during childbirth. People say that feverfew's pain-relieving effect comes from a biochemical called parthenolides, which stops the blood vessels from getting too big during headaches. The plant can also stop you from getting dizzy, ease the pain of allergies, stop blood clots, and ease the pain of arthritis.

A lot of good research on people has shown that feverfew can help avoid and treat migraines. A study done by the School of Postgraduate Medicine and Health Science in the United Kingdom. compared the outcomes of six different studies. Researchers tested feverfew and found that it does work to stop migraines and doesn't pose any big safety concerns.

You can get feverfew in capsules, pills, and a liquid extract. It should be normal for supplements to have at least 0.2% parthenolide. Fetifew leaves can be used to make tea, but they taste bitter and might make your mouth hurt.

7. St. John's Wort.

For more than 2,000 years, people have used St. John's Wort as a medicine because it can help with depression and pain. It makes a lot of biologically active chemicals, but hypericin and hyperforin are the most useful in medicine. St. John's Wort is useful because it can help with depression, ease the symptoms of PMS, boost happiness during menopause, reduce inflammation, soothe skin irritations, and make OCD symptoms better.

The Institute of Psychological Sciences in the UK did a study with 36 women between the ages of 18 and 45 who had regular periods and were identified with mild PMS. The women were given either 900 milligrams of St. John's Wort tablets or similar tablets that didn't contain any medicine. This went on for two menstrual cycles, and then the doses were switched for the next two cycles. During the study, the women were asked to rate their symptoms every day. They talked about how depressed, angry, hormonally balanced, and hormonally stimulated they felt. The tests showed that St. John's Wort worked better than a sugar pill at helping with the physical and mental signs of PMS.

8. Ginkgo Biloba

Ginkgo biloba, which is also called "maidenhair," is an old plant product that has been used for thousands of years in Traditional Chinese Medicine to treat a wide range of health problems. Recent studies have found a link between it and better brain function. Researchers from Beijing University of Chinese Medicine looked at data from 14 randomized controlled studies that included people who had a brain injury. They found that ginkgo biloba extract improved the neurological impairment and quality of life in nine of the trials.

Ginkgo biloba can also help with memory and focus, lower the risk of dementia and Alzheimer's disease, fight anxiety and depression, keep eyes healthy, ease the symptoms of ADHD, boost libido, and ease the pain of fibromyalgia.

You can get ginkgo biloba in the form of capsules, tablets, liquid extract, and dried leaves. The pure extract form has between 24% and 32% flavonoids and between 6% and 13% terpenoids.

9. Saw Palmetto

Some of the supplements that men with prostate cancer and benign prostatic hyperplasia take the most are saw palmetto pills. It has been shown that saw palmetto lowers the production of the enzyme 5-alpha reductase. This enzyme changes testosterone into DHT, which is an androgen and sex hormone. Men's health problems, like losing their libido, having a swollen prostate, and hair loss, are made worse by DHT. However, DHT is important because it helps men grow and develop.

A study released in 2003 in the journal American Family Physician shows that saw palmetto can help ease the symptoms of benign prostatic hyperplasia. It looked like saw palmetto worked about the same way that drugs like finasteride do, but it was easier to take and cost less.

Saw palmetto can help with conditions caused by DHT, but it can also fight inflammation, boost the immune system, treat lung problems, and make you feel calmer.

10. Aloe Vera

In traditional Indian medicine, aloe vera is used to treat pain, skin problems, worm infestations, and be incontinence. This substance is often suggested for the treatment of fungal diseases in Chinese medicine. In the West, it is widely used in the food, drug, and cosmetics industries. Aloe vera is thought to be the biologically active type of aloe. Surprisingly, more than 75 possibly active parts of the plant have been found, such as enzymes, vitamins, minerals, saccharides, amino acids, anthraquinones, lignin, saponins, and salicylic acids. It gives us 20 of the 22 amino acids we need and all eight of the important amino acids.

Aloe vera has been shown to be cleansing, anti-inflammatory, antiviral, and antifungal in studies. The plant is also good for building up the defense system and has not been linked to any allergies. The Journal of Research in Medical Sciences published a study that found that 33 people with irritable bowel syndrome who took 30 milliliters of aloe vera juice twice a day felt less pain. The participants also had less flatulence, but their stools stayed the same in terms of consistency, urgency, and regularity.

As well as its many health benefits, aloe vera can help soothe rashes and other skin irritations, heal burns and cold sores, keep the skin, hair, and head moist, provide antioxidants, and lower inflammation. Aloe vera can be bought at most health food shops and put on the skin or eaten.

Warnings About Herbal Medicine

The U.S. Dietary Supplement Health and Education Act calls herbal supplements dietary supplements. This means that, unlike prescription drugs, they are not tried to show that they are safe and effective. This is the reason why some companies can sell herbal goods that aren't really herbal. If you want to use herbs as medicine, make sure you buy 100 percent pure goods from a company you can trust. This makes sure that you get the best product possible, one that hasn't been harmed by cheaper fillers or grown with heavy metals or pesticides.

Additionally, herbal medicines can cause allergic reactions or mix badly with common medicines. That is why you should talk to your doctor before starting any herbal treatments. Herbalists, naturopathic doctors, pharmacies, medical doctors, and people who practice Traditional Chinese Medicine can all tell you about herbs and help you decide which herb will help your health the most. When you use a plant, make sure you learn about it on your own and find out if it has any side effects and how much to take.

Last Words on Herbal Medicine

- Products from the natural world have been used for many different reasons throughout history. Herbal medicine has been used for more than 5,000 years, as shown in writing records.

- Botanicals, which are also called herbal drugs, are naturally occurring substances that come from plants and are used to treat illness in traditional healing practices in a certain area.

- Today, herbalism is known for focusing on health and happiness in general rather than just treating illness or disease as it happens.

- Herbal medicine is easy to get, cheaper, and has some of the same health benefits as modern drugs.

- Turmeric, saw palmetto, St. John's Wort, and aloe vera are some of the most well-known and widely used plants.

- Research shows that herbal products may have fewer negative side effects than regular medicines, but it's still important for people to choose clean, high-quality products. Before you start using herbal products for a long time, you should talk to a health care worker or herbalist.

How can herbal medicines and remedies make my life better?

Herbal medicine can help you feel better and make your life better in general.

More and more people are interested in holistic health. A lot of people are starting to understand the good things that can happen when you use herbs. Different herbs can help you in different ways, depending on what you need.

You need to find herbs and plants that are right for you. Like, the herbs that will give you more energy might not be the same ones that will help your cough.

How to Choose the Best Herbal Medicines for You

1. What plants and herbs do I need?

A lot of different herbs and plants are good for you in their own ways. If you're not sure, talk to a skilled doctor.

Some herbs can help with different kinds of sickness. Recipes are different based on what you need:

Anxiety: If you're feeling stressed, try a mix of Chai Hu Shu Gan San. This mixture has Bupleurum Chinese (chai hu), Cyperus rotundus (xiang fu), and Cnidium (chuan xiong). It can help with liver qi (life force or vital energy) that is stuck. Gan Mai Da Zao Tang is another one you can try if you have a heart problem. It is made up of Chinese jujubes (da zao), licorice root (gan cao), and wheat grain (xiao mai).

Flu: If you want to get better faster while you're sick, try Yin Qiao San (warm symptoms, like heat). It's an old recipe that uses herbs that lower fever, like honeysuckle (jin–yin hua), forsythia fruit (lian qiao), burdock seed (niu bang zi), or Gui Zhi Tang (chills). Sang Ju Yin, which has chrysanthemum flower (ju hua) and mulberry leaf (sang ye), might help with a cough or sore throat. Sha Shen Mai Dong Tang can help with lung yin shortage, which means the lungs aren't getting enough support, which can cause coughs, sore throats, and other problems. Glehnia (sha shen) and Ophiopogon (mai dong) make up this mixture.

Anemia: If you have anemia, the best foods for you are red dates, goji berries, longan, and codonopsis root (dang shen). The best way to use these is to make plant teas. Chrysanthemum and goji berries can be brewed together to get rid of liver heat, which shows up as red eyes.

2. How to Get the Most Out of Herbal Medicine

Talk to your doctor to make sure that none of the medicines you are already taking will affect your herbal medicines. This is what you should do to get the most out of your natural vitamins.

Always make sure you are following the directions for getting ready. Depending on how you eat them, some herbs can help you in different ways.

3. How to Get Your Herbal Medicine Ready and Keep It Safe

Doctor Lim says that you should always keep your herbs somewhere cool and dry. The herbs can also be kept in the fridge to make them last longer. Some raw herbs may be ground into a powder and put into capsules so they can be taken directly. Some have to be brewed in order to get their healing qualities out, while others can be done with ethanol. Someone who sells herbs or the store where you buy them can tell you more about them.

Some flowers that are seeds will need to be crushed before they can be boiled. When flowers or leaves float in water, you should put them in different bags to make things easier to handle. Peppermint leaves and other herbs that lose their flavor quickly should only be added to the pot just before the heat is turned off.

4. More than just pills, powders, capsules, and teas

There are different ways to take plant medicine, such as in capsule form for easier use.

When it comes to medical herbs, there are a lot of different ways to take them. Some treatments are pastes, soaks, topical medicines, and things you can eat, drink, or mix with other things (like food, teas, decoctions, granules, tablets, and capsules).

Doctor Lim also says you should try plant soups. Superior Nurturing Soup is one of her suggestions. It's good for people of all ages and helps those who aren't hungry or who are bloated. She also says that people with a weak immune system or who are recovering from surgery or disease should eat Lingzhi Tonic Soup. Last but not least, she suggests Si Shen Soup and Vitality Tonic Soup for people who need more energy. Do talk to a professional before you try the soups.

How to Get Healthier

It's normal to not see or feel effects right away when you're trying to improve your health and wellness. It may seem hard to improve your health and wellness, but if you make small changes every day, you will start to see benefits in no time. Do not rush into anything when you are learning about plant medicine. Take your time and learn what your body and mind need to be healthy and balanced.

How to Grow, Gather, and Store Herbs

Herbs are simple to grow and aren't usually hurt by bugs or diseases. For the average family, a few short rows of herbs in a flower or vegetable yard will be enough. It's easy to keep herbs fresh and store them for up to a year.

There are three types of herbs: annual, biennial, and permanent. Remember this as you look for them in the yard. Sort flowers into groups based on how much light and water they need. Herbs do best in dirt that drains well and has a pH between 6.0 and 7.0. They also need four to six hours of sun per day.

Perennial flowers should be planted in a spot that won't be tilled. If you plant herbs that spread by runners, like mint, directly in the yard, you should keep them in pots. Pots should be sunk into the ground so that the top two inches are above the soil. This way, runners can be taken out of the yard before they take root.

Plant and Seed Spreading

You can start herbs inside or outside. There is an easy way to plant small seeds: put them in pots with seed-starting mix about six weeks before the last frost date. Tear-shaped plants like parsley, dill, and cilantro do well in clay pots. You can use vermiculite, moist seed-starting mix, or ground sphagnum moss to cover the seeds. Cut plants in half so that there are four or five in each pot. You can also start bigger seeds in separate pots and then thin them out until you only have one plant left. If you want to grow plants, keep the soil's surface wet.

Cuttings are the best way to grow some herbs, like rosemary and sweet bay. Root cuttings in a 3-inch plastic pot or any other container that works and has holes in it for draining. A mix of perlite and vermiculite works well as a growing medium. Cover the pot with plastic and keep the rooting medium wet. This will keep the humidity high. When plants are young, keep them out of direct sunlight to keep them from dying. Plant the cuttings in dirt after they have grown roots.

Once there is no longer a chance of frost, plant annual herbs outside. During the growth season, get rid of weeds so that plants don't have to compete with them for water and nutrients. An inch of organic mulch will help keep the earth moist and keep weeds from growing.

It's best to water flowers first thing in the morning. The water will get to the roots of the plants more quickly if you water them when it is cooler. To help roots grow, water deeply. During droughts, plants may need to be watered, but once they are established, many herbs are very immune to drought.

Harvesting

Herbs should be picked often during the growing season, when the plant has enough leaves to keep growing. For most plants, cut the stems just above a group of leaves. For parsley and chives, cut the stems at the base. Get rid of any bad or dead leaves and clean off any dirt that might be on them. Spray the leaves with a yard hose the day before you pick them if they are very dirty. Pick the herbs early in the day, before the sun's heat takes away the oils that make them taste good.

If you want to dry herbs, you should pick them right before the flowers open, because that's when the leaves have the most volatile, pungent oils. By late summer, stop picking annual plants' leaves so they have time to store enough carbs for the winter.

You can save seeds to use in cooking or to start plants from. When seeds turn from green to brown or gray, it's time to harvest them. Let them dry completely before putting them away.

How to Keep and Store

Wash and dry the leaves gently so they can be used right away. Keep extras in the cooler of your fridge in plastic bags that aren't sealed. Wash them before you use them.

There are several ways to dry herbs so that you can use them later.

- Let small bunches dry in the air by taking the leaves off the bottom 2 inches of the stem. Use a rubber band to hold the stems in place because they will shrink as they dry. Hold the bunches up in a dark, well-ventilated space that is free of dust. Mark each bunch because dried herbs tend to look the same. The best results happen when the leaves dry quickly without using heat or being in the sun. If you want to keep the color and oils in thick, juicy leaves like basil, you may need to dry them quickly in a warm oven, dehydrator, or sun dryer.

- If the leaves aren't too small, they can be taken off the stems and dried side by side on trays made of window screens or 1-inch-mesh hardware cloth that is safe for food. Once or twice a day, gently stir the leaves to help them dry faster. Note that the screen should be safe for food. An old screen may be made of a metal that reacts with light.

- You can dry things in the oven at low heat (110°F or less) by leaving the door slightly open. Place the leaves on a cookie sheet and stir them every so often.

- A dehydrator is a good choice for drying a lot of herbs at once. Set the temperature on the dehydrator to between 95°F and 115°F to warm it up. Make sure the herbs don't touch or cross when you put them on the dehydrator tray. If you need to, you can put a fine, food-grade plastic screen over the dehydrator tray to keep the herbs from going to the bottom. Take out some of the trays to make room for the bigger leaves. Dry leaves on the lowest setting possible for the best taste. If there is no thermostat on the dehydrator, set it to the smallest time possible. Cut the roots into ¼- to ½-inch pieces and dry them. Roots need six to ten hours to dry fully. When they are, they will be stiff.

- Herb leaves are dry when they break easily when you rub them together. You can use a rolling pin, a fine mesh sieve, a mixer, or a mortar and pestle to break up the leaves into a powder or ground form. Keep the leaves whole and crush them when you're ready to add them to food to keep the flavor.

- Keep dried herbs in a cool, dry place out of direct sunlight in containers that won't let air in. If you store the herbs the right way, they will keep their flavors and vital oils for up to a year. There are several ways to freeze flowers. Pick the method based on what you plan to do with the herb in the kitchen.

- Fill an ice cube tray with chopped clean herbs mixed with either water or oil, based on what you plan to use them for. Go ahead and freeze it. Once the cubes are frozen, put them back in the freezer in a bag or jar that is made to handle freezing. Always write the date and what's in each jar or bag on the label. Whether you use a neutral-tasting canola oil or a stronger olive oil depends on your personal taste and what goes best with the herb's flavor and strength.

- Put clean, dry leaves on a cookie sheet in a single layer and freeze them. When the herbs are frozen, quickly put them in a freezer bag or jar with a note so they don't thaw. When leaves are frozen in this way, they shouldn't stick together, making it easy to take out the amount that is needed.

- If you want to freeze herbs, sealed glass jars are better than plastic cases because they keep the smell inside.

- Rosemary, thyme, and dill are some herbs that freeze well on their stems. Put a few stems in a freezer bag or wrap them in aluminum foil and then stick them in the bag. A label.

- Herbs will change shape when frozen, but their taste will stay the same if you do it right. You can pickle dill weed that has been thawed, but it will look darker and be less stiff. Herbs should not be thawed before being used in cooking. You can add them straight from the freezer to stews and soups or to the pan. You have one year to use frozen veggies.

Getting bigger in pots and inside

Herbs like trailing rosemary, variegated sage, oregano, and chives look great in outdoor containers and are a quick and easy way to grow herbs when you don't have much room in your yard. When you plant things in pots, use good potting soil. Garbage or yard soil should not be used. Making sure the pot has holes for draining is important. Also, don't put rocks or broken pottery in the bottom of the pot. Plants in the ground take longer to dry out than plants in containers, so make sure to water them often. You can grow most small herb plants inside. If you grow them in the sun, away from drafts and heat sources, you can use the leaves for cooking all winter long. Basil, oregano, rosemary, thyme, and parsley are some of the best ones to try. If the pot has a bowl, remove any extra water that is collecting under it as soon as you water the plant.

Uses

Adding herbs to food is a good way to make it taste better. When you add herbs to recipes, keep in mind that dried herbs have more oil than fresh herbs. For every teaspoon of dried herbs, use two tablespoons of fresh ones. Sheaths with pleasant smells aren't the only things that use herbs. Potpourri, candles, soaps, and cosmetics also use them.

Chapter 3

Natural Remedies For Everyday Illnesses

Natural remedies for cough and sore throat

- Tea: licorice and slippery elm are two ingredients in some teas that coat the throat and help soothe discomfort.

- Honey: can help soothe sore throats and stop coughing because it coats the throat. You can eat it with a spoon or mix it into tea.

- Echinacea: can shorten the time that cold symptoms last, especially if you take it in the first two or three days. You can get it as tea, drops, or pills.

- Elderberry syrup: this syrup can help with colds and flu because it fights viruses. Do what it says on the package.

- Pelargonium: is a plant that is used in some herbal cough and cold pills. It cuts down on the length and intensity of colds.

**Try each one by itself to see which one you like best. Don't use all three at the same time.

Digestive home remedies

- Ginger: can help with stomachaches, motion sickness, and feeling sick. You can drink ginger tea (look for medical brands) or snack on candied ginger when you're out and about.

- Probiotics: These are probiotics, which are living yeasts and bacteria that are good for your skin. When you have diarrhea because of an illness or antibiotic use, probiotics can help. It can be found in foods and products like yogurt, miso paste, kombucha, kimchi, and **raw sauerkraut.**

Topical medicines for pain and skin discomfort

- Arnica cream helps with body aches, pains, and bruises.
- For bacterial or fungal diseases, tea tree oil can help reduce swelling. You can use it to treat acne and athlete's foot on the spot.
- Calendula: calms skin problems like diaper rash and acne.

Natural ways to help you sleep

- Tea: As you wind down in the evening, try chamomile tea.
- Lavender oil is used in aromatherapy to help people calm down and rest. Safe for both little kids and older people.

Natural ways to deal with stress

- Take five minutes to breathe slowly and deeply before you start your day. Think about the people in your life, the day ahead, and what you're thankful for.
- Teach your kids different ways to breathe on the way to school to help them get ready for the day. Take four-second breaths in and six-second breaths out to slow down your breathing. This turns on the part of our nervous system that makes us feel calm.
- Pick music that makes you feel good to listen to on your way to and from school or work.

- Take a few minutes to get ready for the trip home after work. Put the problems at work to rest and turn your attention to your family.

To be safe, let your doctor know about any herbal medicines or vitamins you are taking. If you are pregnant, nursing, or taking prescription drugs, talk to your doctor before adding herbal remedies to your routine.

Help from Natural Remedies

The good news is that there are many natural alternatives that will not only help heal small cuts and bruises but will also make your bathroom more spacious. Some people may not believe that natural remedies work, but in the last few decades, science progress has shown that plant-based cures aren't just old wives' tales.

Natural remedies, or medicines made from plants and herbs, have been used for thousands of years, long before there were neighborhood drug stores. Back then, there were fruit trees, honeybees, and herb gardens. You've probably used one of these before: herbal teas for a cold, essential oils for a headache, or plant-based vitamins to help you sleep.

However, herbal supplements can have strong effects or combine badly with regular medicines, so do not try to diagnose yourself. People who already have health problems or who are pregnant or nursing should always talk to their doctor before trying natural treatments.

These are some of our favorites that are great for coughs, cuts, and bruises.

Lavender to sleep with

This pleasant "garden" smell can help with nervousness and insomnia, and lavender essential oil is not only strong, but also well-known for its benefits. It has been shown that a few drops in a warm bath or humidifier can help people fall asleep and sleep better. So, it helps with worry, depression, and mood swings. Lavender also calms the skin, making it less red and helping scars heal. It also improves skin tone by increasing blood flow. If you put it on a mosquito bite, the itching will go away.

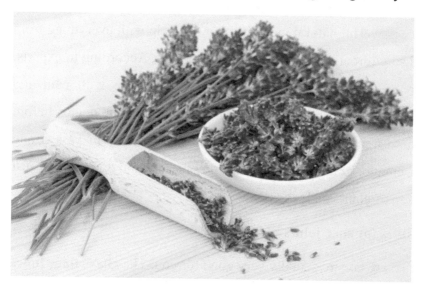

Baking soda for making things swell

This is in a lot of over-the-counter meds and can help with pain and infections. It can help with rashes by reducing swelling and itching. It can also help with cuts, scrapes, burns, bug stings, and mouth ulcers. Before bed, put it on a small cut or scrape in your mouth. When you wake up, it won't hurt.

Mint helps your body digest food.

Mint is often used to treat stomach pain, and it can also help pregnant women who are sick with morning sickness. It works by turning on the enzymes that break down food. Additionally, mint can help clear up stuffy noses, throats, and lungs if you have a cold that keeps coming back. This natural remedy also helps soothe sore throats caused by coughing because it kills germs.

Ginger for sickness

Ginger is a powerful natural medicine that can help with everything from colds and sore throats to sickness and feeling sick. According to experts, eating up to 4 grams of ginger every day may help with pain and inflammation. However, you should always talk to your doctor before using natural treatments along with regular medicine. To make a strong medicine, chop or grate this superfood into sauces, salad dressings, or just put it on top of your salad.

Green chilies for sore joints

Peppers that are hot are actually very good for you. They have three times as much vitamin C as oranges. Also, they are full of vitamins A, B, and E. Studies show that ginger, chili, and other spices can help lower inflammation. Capsaicin, the chemical that gives tomatoes and peppers their heat, works on pain by making the skin hot and then numb. This helps with sore muscles. That's why it's used to treat joint pain as a cream or a patch on the skin.

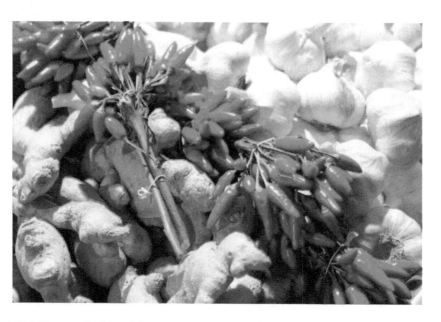

Garlic can help with many health problems.

In the past, garlic was put on wounds to help them heal and keep them from getting infected. Garlic is known to fight germs, viruses, fungi, and even parasites. Over the years, it has been used to treat fevers, asthma, high blood pressure, liver problems, gas, rheumatism, and diabetes. Studies show that eating one to two raw cloves a day may be good for you, but there aren't any government suggestions.

Reishi Mushroom to calm down

People are now using these mushrooms to lower their high blood pressure and cholesterol. Reishi is a famous fungus in Eastern medicine for boosting the immune system. However, if you take reishi along with blood pressure medications, your blood pressure may drop too low. Reishi has also been used in old Chinese and Japanese ceremonies as a natural way to help people calm down before bed. So, if you've been tired, make some warm tea to drink before going to sleep.

For a cold, steam is good.

You might have tried cough syrup or lost sleep from constantly fluffing up your pillows to get rid of that annoying cough. But steam is the easy answer to getting rid of a cough. Austrian researchers found that people who constantly use saunas get colds less often. It's good for you to breathe in warm air in the shower. Or, put some eucalyptus oil in a bowl of hot water and put a towel over your head as you lower it over the bowl. Then, close your eyes and take in the soothing scents.

Health Benefits of Healing Herbs

It is either illegal to pick healing herbs from the wild or on purpose so that they can be used as medicine or to heal people. Herbal medicines can be made from the leaves, bark, stems, roots, seeds, and/or flowers of a plant.

When it comes to healing plants, there is some proof that they can treat or ease the symptoms of certain health problems. Some examples are

- ashwagandha
- Rosemary
- Elechinacea
- Onion
- Orange Ginger
- Ginger
- Ginger
- Rosemary
- St. John's Wort
- Turmeric

It talks about how these healing plants have been used in the past, what study has found about them, how to take them, and things to think about.

Do not forget that herbal medicines are not miracle cures for everything that is wrong with you. They can help as extra treatments. Also, they can have risks and side effects, and the Food and Drug Administration (FDA) doesn't keep an eye on their safety or effectiveness.

ashwagandha

The plant Withania somnifera is where ashwagandha comes from. This plant is also called Indian ginseng and Indian winter cherry. The shrub grows naturally in Africa and Asia. It can also be found in some places of the Middle East and India.

Uses in the past

People have used ashwagandha for thousands of years because it is good for you. In Ayurvedic medicine, which is India's traditional method of medicine, the herb is often used to increase energy, lower stress and anxiety, and ease pain and inflammation.

Researchers have found that this strong plant lowers cortisol levels by a large amount, which helps lower stress and anxiety.1 It is known as an adaptogen, which means it helps protect against stress.2

As well as improving male sexual health, ashwagandha is said to help with erectile dysfunction, boost drive (sexual desire), and make sexual pleasure better. This is because the herb can raise testosterone levels in men.

Getting ready

Ashwagandha is a food supplement that comes in capsule, tincture, and powder forms. Ashwagandha powder can taste earthy and bitter, so it works best when mixed with something else, like coffee, tea, smoothies, or sweets. In the past, it was mixed with water, honey, or ghee.

Add a quarter to a half teaspoon of ashwagandha powder to hot drinks or soups. Even though it can be taken at any time, it works best when taken about 30 minutes before a meal.

Most people don't feel the benefits of ashwagandha right away. It might take a few weeks to notice that ashwagandha is helping you.

Think about it

Ashwagandha is safe for most people to use. Some of the most common side effects are sleepiness, stomach pain, and diarrhea. Anticonvulsants, benzodiazepines, and barbiturates are just a few of the medicines that people who take them shouldn't take. The plant may combine with these drugs.

If you are pregnant, don't take ashwagandha because high amounts can cause you to lose the baby.

Chamomile flower

The chamomile flower comes from India, Asia, and Western Europe. Now, it can grow anywhere in the United States. There are two kinds of chamomile: Roman, which grows all year and smells like apples, and German, which grows in the Midwest.

Uses in the past

In the United States, chamomile is a famous herbal remedy that is often used to calm down and feel better. As a tea, chamomile is "likely safe," says the National Center for Complementary and Integrative Health, which is part of the National Institutes of Health. It might also be safe to take by mouth for a short time. We don't know enough about how safe it is to use chamomile as medicine over a long period of time.

While in Europe, chamomile is used to help wounds heal and lower swelling and redness. This herbal remedy is very famous, and it has been shown to work.

A 2016 review said that chamomile can be used in many ways. It's often used for its antibacterial, antidepressant, anti-inflammatory, anti-diarrheal, and antioxidant properties. It can also help with osteoarthritis in the knee, ulcerative colitis, premenstrual syndrome, and other digestive problems.

Getting ready

You can make chamomile tea, put it on as a rub, or put it on your skin to soothe it. To smell and taste, chamomile tea is like apple cider. To get the tea ready:

1. As you boil water, add 1 teaspoon of dried flowers to each cup.
2. Put the flower petals in a tea strainer.
3. Boil water and pour it over the flowers.
4. Let it sit for five minutes.

If you want a cooler drink, you can add ice to the tea. In most health food shops, you can buy chamomile as a tea or in capsule form. If you use capsules, make sure they are made by a medicinal company. It's possible that grades like therapeutic marks aren't as good.

Think about it

Chamomile may make people with allergies sick, and some have even died from anaphylaxis, which is a serious allergic reaction that occurs all over the body. If you take blood thinners or the drug cyclosporine to fight rejection, don't use chamomile. It might not work well with these medicines.

A plant called Echinacea

It is an ornamental plant in the same family as daisies. In early to late summer, the flower's big pink petals open up. Echinacea grows in eastern and central North America. The leaf, stalk, and root are all widely used in medicine.

Uses in the past

Echinacea has been used for a long time to treat toothaches, bowel problems, snake bites, seizures, skin irritations, arthritis, and even cancer. In modern times, echinacea is often used as a home treatment to shorten or stop the flu and colds. A lot of people also use it to help wounds heal.

A lot of the chemicals in echinacea are thought to help with pain relief, reducing inflammation, fighting viruses, and protecting cells from damage.

Some studies show that using echinacea to stop upper respiratory infections might be a little helpful. But more research is needed to find out if it really works to stop or shorten the length of a cold.

Getting ready

You can get echinacea in the form of capsules, tinctures, and tea (both bagged and loose-leaf). There is no set amount of echinacea that should be taken every day. How to make echinacea tea with loose leaves:

1. Fill a mug with tea, flowers, and leaves.
2. Bring water to a boil and pour 8 ounces into the mug.
3. For up to 15 minutes, let the tea steep.
4. Strain to get the plant parts out.
5. Add honey, stevia, or other natural sweeteners to taste.

Think about it

Echinacea can be hard on the stomach and may make you feel sick. Experts say that you should only use Echinacea for a short time. When used for eight weeks or more, it can hurt the nervous system and liver.

Before you use Echinacea, talk to your doctor or nurse. It could change how your medicines work, especially medicines that affect your liver.

Are you allergic to plants in the same family as daisies, like ragweed, marigolds, or daisies? If so, you might be allergic to Echinacea.

Garlic

Garlic is an annual plant that comes from Central Asia. It is grown for its tasty bulbs. It is now grown all over the world by many nations. People value garlic for both its culinary uses and its health benefits.

Uses in the past

Garlic has been used by people for a very long time. In traditional medicine, it was used to stop infections, lower blood pressure, treat tuberculosis, colic, liver disease, and intestine worms, and bring down fevers.

Garlic contains chemicals that kill germs, fight cancer, and reduce inflammation. Garlic has been shown to lower blood pressure and lower the risk of having a heart attack or stroke.

Some types of cancer might be easier to avoid if you eat garlic. It has been found that eating cooked or raw garlic on a regular basis may lower the chance of colorectal cancer.

Getting ready

You can eat garlic either raw or cooked. You can also use the powder to season soups, stews, meats, and veggies.

You can get garlic vitamins in the form of capsules, oil, and tincture. The daily amounts you should take depend on how you are using garlic, such as:

- about 2 to 5 grams of raw, fresh garlic
- about 0.4 to 1.2 grams of garlic powder, dried
- Two to five milligrams of garlic oil
- Water with 2,400 mg of garlic extract

Think about it

Talk to your doctor before taking garlic as a vitamin because it is good for you. If you are on blood thinners, you shouldn't eat garlic because it can make you more likely to bleed. This is also why you shouldn't eat a lot of garlic before surgery or the dentist.

Ginger

The stem of ginger (Zingiber officinale) is bushy, and the flowers are yellow-green. Ginger is in the Zingiberaceae family and comes from Asia and India. The flexible spice comes from the ginger plant's underground stem and is used all over the world in drinks and foods.

The fresh rhizoma (root stem) of Zingiber officinale Roscoe is used in traditional Chinese medicine. It is known as Zingiberis Rhizoma Recens.

Uses in the past

Ginger has been used in many ancient medicines around the world since the 1500s. Ginger was so valuable and sought after for its health benefits more than 2,000 years ago that a pound of it was worth the price of a cow.

People used it to treat common illnesses like sickness, pain, and throwing up. Ginger is unique because it is now considered a plant, a food, and a medicine.

When it comes to health benefits, ginger is probably best known for its ability to help people who are sick feel better. Researchers have confirmed that ginger may help people who are sick during surgery or during pregnancy feel better when they feel like throwing up. Ginger may also help with nausea caused by treatment.

Ginger can also help with pain because it reduces inflammation and protects cells from damage. In one study, ginger helped people with osteoarthritis feel less pain and move around better.

Getting ready

Ginger comes in a lot of different forms, such as fresh, dried, pickled, roasted, and powdered. It smells strong and hot, and it tastes sweet and spicy at the same time. In most grocery shops, ground ginger root is what you can find on the spice shelves. It's often used for baking and cooking.

Ginger can be drunk in many different ways, such as in tea. Most food stores sell ginger tea bags, or you can use fresh ginger to make your own at home. Peel the skin off of fresh ginger with a vegetable knife before you eat it.

Think about it

Ginger may also be safe to use on the skin, but it is thought to be safe to take by mouth as a food supplement. Side effects are usually mild and include diarrhea, heartburn, and stomach pain, especially when taken in large amounts.

Ginger is safe to use during pregnancy, but if you want to stop feeling sick and throwing up during pregnancy, talk to your doctor before you start.

Gingko

Ginkgo biloba, which is just called "ginkgo," is one of the oldest tree species that is still alive. Ginkgo is one of the most popular plant medicines in the US. It comes from Asia. Extracts, pills, and tablets are all made from ginkgo leaves.

You can also make tea out of ginkgo leaves. Chinese medicine also uses the nut to help people who wheeze.

Uses in the past

For thousands of years, ginkgo leaves have been used as medicine. Some of these are managing tinnitus (ringing in the ears), bronchitis, asthma, and chronic fatigue. There are some people who think that ginkgo can really help your brain, but more research is needed to be sure.

The National Center for Complementary and Integrative Health says there isn't strong proof that ginkgo can help with any health problem.

Getting ready

You can buy gingko in the form of capsules, tablets, liquid extract, and dried leaves or tea. At this time, there is no standard dose of ginkgo that is suggested. In different research projects, different amounts and types of drugs have been used.

The right amount for you will depend on your age, health history, sex, and the kind of medicine being used. In general, it's better to start with a smaller number until you find the right one for you. It could be up to six weeks before you feel better after taking ginkgo.

Think about it

If you take a supplement, make sure that it is made from only oils of ginkgo leaves. There is a poison in the seeds that can make people have seizures. Headaches, stomachaches, dizziness, and allergic responses are some of the side effects.

Ginkgo may make you more likely to bleed. Due to possible drug reactions, it shouldn't be taken with NSAIDs, blood thinners, seizure medicines, or tricyclic antidepressants.

Ginseng

There are many health benefits said to come from the root ginseng. There are many kinds of ginseng. One type is called "man-root" because it looks like a person.

Panax quinquefolius, or American ginseng, is a perennial herb that grows in deciduous woods in the United States. Panax ginseng, which is also known as Asian ginseng, comes from China, Korea, and eastern Siberia. The plant name Panax comes from the word "panacea," which means "all-purpose" and refers to ginseng's many medical uses.

The plant Eleutherococcus senticosus, which grows in Siberia, is also known as eleuthero or ci wu jia in traditional Chinese medicine. It works more like an adaptogen and is not as strong as the other types. Panax notoginseng, which is also known as radix notoginseng or sanchi, has been used for a long time to stop bleeding.

Uses in the past

Ginseng has been used in traditional Chinese treatment for a very long time. Some of the health benefits of this plant are that it fights inflammation, cancer, obesity, and viruses. This is why it is still used as medicine.

Ginseng is thought to help the blood flow, boost the immune system, and lower the risk of some kinds of cancer. It has also been shown that the strong herb can lower blood sugar and make diabetes therapy better.

Studies have shown that ginseng can help people learn and remember things better. Because of this, it is often used as an anti-aging herb to help older people keep their brains healthy.25 Ginseng has also been shown to reduce inflammation in the body and is just as good at relieving pain and inflammation as nonsteroidal anti-inflammatory (NSAID) drugs.

Getting ready

Ginseng can be eaten in a lot of different ways to get its health benefits. When you buy fresh ginseng, you can eat it either raw or cooked. You can also make tea with freshly cut ginseng. You can also add it to food, and stir-fry and soups enjoy it a lot. But if you buy expensive ginseng, these food uses will cost you too much.

As a dietary supplement, you can also find ginseng in some drug shops and health food stores. It comes in capsule, powder, and extract types that you can buy.

At this time, there is no daily suggested amount of ginseng. Different amounts have been looked at in studies, ranging from 0.5 to 3 grams of fresh ginseng and 100 to 800 mg of extract. Follow the advice on the bottle for how much ginseng to take.

Think about it

Ginseng is usually safe to take and doesn't have any major side effects. Headaches, stomachaches, and trouble sleeping are some of the most common side effects.

Some evidence suggests that taking ginseng for a long time makes it less effective, so only take it for two to three weeks at a time, with a break of one to two weeks in between.

If you take diabetes medicine, make sure you keep a close eye on your glucose levels while you're taking ginseng to make sure they don't drop too low.

If you are taking any medicines, talk to your doctor before taking ginseng as a supplement. Do not take ginseng if you have a condition that makes you bleed easily or if you are taking blood thinners like Coumadin (warfarin).

Lavender

Lavender (Lavandula) is an evergreen shrub that grows in low mounds and has a pleasant smell. It is one of the most famous herbs in the world. It comes from the mint family and does well in many places around the world.

This herb is very useful and has been studied a lot because it might be good for your health. It is used in personal care items, baking, and essential oils.

Uses in the past

Lavender has been used by people for hundreds of years in everything from perfumes to massage to medicine. In the past, people used the herb's healing qualities to clean wounds, treat insect bites and burns, and keep them from getting some diseases.

Lavender may help you sleep, remember things better, ease pain, and feel better overall. Lavender has been shown to help with seizures, fight free radicals, reduce inflammation, and kill germs in both animal and human tests.

There are many medical and therapeutic uses for lavender, which is a powerful plant. Due to its cooling effects, lavender essential oil may help ease stress and help you get a good night's sleep.31

Researchers have also found that the essential oil can ease pain. It may help with headaches, back pain, arthritis pain, and menstrual cramps.

Getting ready

Lavender comes in a lot of different forms, such as powder, dried flower, and essential oil. You can grow lavender in your yard if you live in a place where it can do well. Because it smells good, lavender is often used in perfumes, shampoos, and creams and lotions.

You can use an air diffuser to spread the essential oil or rub it directly into your skin after mixing it with a carrier oil like olive or almond oil. You can also put it on your sheets or a cotton ball and breathe it in for perfume.

You can buy lavender tea in tea bags already made, or you can soak dried lavender flower buds in hot water to make a tea that doesn't have any caffeine.

Think about it

Some people may be allergic to lavender essential oil or have skin irritations when they use it. Before putting the essential oil on your skin, you should always mix it with a carrier oil. If you get a headache, feel sick, or throw up after using it, stop using it right away. If you put lavender essential oil in your mouth, it could be harmful.

Lavender taken by mouth, like in a tea, can make you constipated, give you headaches, or make you hungry.

St. John's Wort

The flower of Saint-John's-wort is yellow. It comes from Europe, Western Asia, and North Africa, but it now grows all over the United States. The flower and leaf are used to make plant supplements and medicines that can be used instead of medicine for a number of health problems.

Uses in the past

Saint-John's-wort has been used as medicine for thousands of years to treat a wide range of conditions, such as sadness, insomnia, wound healing, and problems with the kidneys and lungs.

These days, Saint-John's-wort is mostly known as a herbal treatment for sadness. Studies have shown that if used for 12 weeks, it may help people with mild to moderate sadness.

Saint-John's Wort is also used to treat skin problems, obsessive-compulsive disorder (OCD), and to ease the signs of menopause. It can be put on wounds to help them heal and ease muscle pain.

Getting ready

You can get Saint-John's-wort in pills, tinctures, elixirs, and oil or liquid forms, such as oil or liquid. Different supplements may have different strengths and each product will come in a different amount. There isn't enough information to give a normal dose of Saint-John's-wort.

The right amount of Saint-John's-wort for you will depend on your age, gender, and health background. The best people to work with are your doctor, pharmacist, and/or a natural health practitioner. They can tailor your amount to make sure it works and is safe.

Think about it

If you take a lot of Saint-John's Wort, you might become sensitive to sunlight. Before using this plant remedy, talk to your doctor or nurse. It can cause dangerous side effects when taken with some medicines. If you are taking antidepressants, you should not take Saint-John's Wort because it may cause a dangerous rise in serotonin levels.

Turmeric

Turmeric is an annual herbaceous plant that comes from South Asia. It is in the ginger family. For more than 4,000 years, people have used it as medicine.

Uses in the past

A lot of research has been done on turmeric. It can fight cancer, destroy free radicals, reduce inflammation, and kill germs. In Ayurveda and other traditional medical methods, it is used to treat skin problems, lung infections, and digestive problems.

Ayurvedic Health Care

Ayurveda is an Indian traditional medicine system that uses herbs as a main part of its treatments. Herbs are used to keep the heart, body, and mind in balance.

People still like to use turmeric as a natural medicine. People say it can help with allergies, arthritis, digestive problems, respiratory infections, sadness, and liver disease.

According to research, turmeric may be good for your skin whether you take it as a supplement or put it on your face. Turmeric has also been shown to help ease the pain of arthritis in the joints. People who took 100 milligrams of turmeric powder every day had less joint pain, according to one study.

Getting ready

People all over the world use turmeric in their food. You can get turmeric pills in the form of capsules that are made from the dried rhizome, which is the underground stem. People with certain skin conditions can put turmeric paste on their face.

The right amount of turmeric to take depends on what it will be used for. A lot of studies use daily amounts of turmeric between 500 and 2,000 milligrams. How much you take will rely on your age, medical history, sex, and what you want to use it for.

Some people feel a lot better when they take smaller doses, so start with a small amount and see what dose works best for you.

Think about it

Most people think it's safe to eat turmeric in food, take it as a supplement, or put it on their skin in the suggested amounts. Curcumin is an active ingredient in turmeric. Supplements have higher concentrations of curcumin than foods. Taking large amounts of curcumin may upset your stomach and lead to diarrhea, skin rashes, yellow stools, and headaches.

Before taking a turmeric pill, talk to your doctor or nurse. Some prescription drugs and other herbal treatments may not work well with it.

Turmeric can make blood thinners work worse, which raises your chance of bleeding. A review found that turmeric may not work well with some drugs, like antidepressants, blood thinners, antibiotics, chemotherapy drugs, and antihistamines.

Who the FDA Is in Charge of Herbs

The FDA keeps an eye on side effects reported by customers and regulates dietary supplements and food ingredients. You can use the U.S. to report any side effects or safety issues. Safety Reporting Portal for Health and Human Services.

In short

Plants have been used to treat illness, pain, and sickness for thousands of years. Herbs that are good for you come in many forms, such as supplements, tinctures, drinks, and essential oils.

The scientific proof for different herbal remedies is very mixed. Sometimes there is a lot of knowledge and sometimes there isn't much.

Do as much study as you can on any remedies you want to use before you take them to find out what side effects they might have as well as what health benefits they say they can give you.

Chapter 4

How to Make an Herbal Tea Infusion & Decoction

It might be fastest and most effective to make herbal medicine in the form of teas and decoctions. They are an important part of extracting herbs, and learning how to make them should be one of the first things any prospective herbalist does. Within this book, we will talk about the right methods and techniques for making good tea. For those who want to learn more, we will also talk about the chemistry and physical processes of extraction. This will help you understand why we recommend certain steps for making tea and decoction.

How It Works:

When you make a tea or stew, all you're doing is using water to get chemicals from herbs that dissolve in water. Phytochemicals, which are chemicals found in plants, include carbs, enzymes, mucilage, pectins, saponins, flavonoids, and polysaccharides. They can dissolve in water. By breaking up glands and cells that hold more antioxidants, hot water makes the extraction process even better. Some phytochemicals, like most lipids and many alkaloids, don't dissolve in water. This is why tinctures, oil infusions, and other plant preparations are useful. But for the vast majority of plant needs, teas are a perfectly fine, if not pleasant, way to use and enjoy herbs.

What's the Difference Between a Decoction and an Infusion?

One simple difference between infusions (like teas) and decoctions is that decoctions are cooked over low heat while infusions are soaked. This is because some parts of the plant have stronger cell walls and need a little more "coaxing" to get the chemicals we're interested in out of them. For this reason, the softer parts of the plant, like leaves, flowers, and stems, are usually used for drinks. Because these herbs have "softer" cell walls, they break down easily, letting water into the cells. Also, adding boiling water to oil glands that hold essential oils and other aromatic substances can often easily break them open.

Roots, bark, berries, and seeds often have cells that are a lot stronger. To break down cell walls, the materials often need to be simmered (covered) for a long time. To get the many polysaccharides that are in mushrooms, they often need to be decocted as well.

Of course, there are times when these rules don't apply. For instance, marshmallow root is best made by cold soaking because its polysaccharides are easy to get out with just cold water. The chemicals of interest are broken down by hot water, which makes the extraction less effective. Valerian is also a root. But in this case, a hot water mixture is better than a decoction for getting the volatile oils out. On this occasion, letting the root boil can lead to the loss of the volatile oils that help it relax. In short, you usually decoct mushrooms, roots, berries, seeds, barks, and the stems and leaves of plants. To be sure, though, talk to a herbalist, read a good herbal book, or look at the images below.

How to Steep Something:

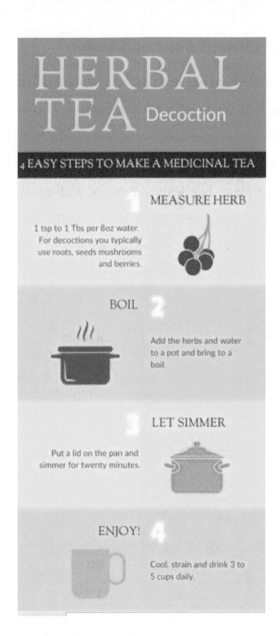

HERBAL TEA Decoction

4 EASY STEPS TO MAKE A MEDICINAL TEA

1 MEASURE HERB

1 tsp to 1 Tbs per 8oz water. For decoctions you typically use roots, seeds mushrooms and berries.

BOIL 2

Add the herbs and water to a pot and bring to a boil.

3 LET SIMMER

Put a lid on the pan and simmer for twenty minutes.

ENJOY! 4

Cool, strain and drink 3 to 5 cups daily.

1. Measure the plant

1 to 3 teaspoons for every 8 ounces of water. If you are using fresh herbs, double the amount of herbs because they contain more water than dried

51

herbs and can water down your broth. You can get better drainage if you grind, crush, or powder the herbs before you decoct them.

2. Bring up to a boil

Fill a pan with cold water. If you put the herbs right into hot water, it might be hard to get the other plant parts out. Add the herbs and bring the water to a boil.

3. Let it Simmer

Put the lid on the pan and let it cook for twenty minutes.

If you want to make a tea mix with both the woodsy and soft parts of a plant, do the following:

- Boil the woody leaves,
- When you take the pot off the heat, add the rest of the herbs. With the lid on, let all the herbs steep for 20 minutes.

4. Have fun!

Let it cool down, then drain and drink. Keep leftovers in the fridge and eat them within a week.

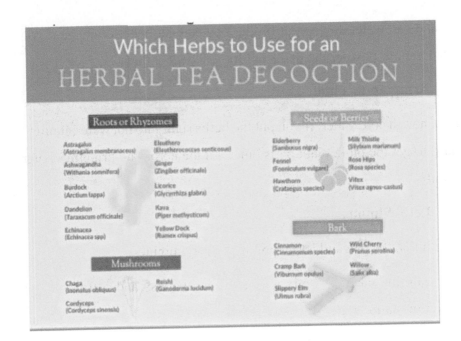

Which Herbs to Use for an HERBAL TEA DECOCTION

Roots or Rhyzomes

Astragalus (Astragalus membranaceus)

Ashwagandha (Withania somnifera)

Burdock (Arctium lappa)

Dandelion (Taraxacum officinale)

Echinacea (Echinacea spp)

Eleuthero (Eleutherococcus senticosus)

Ginger (Zingiber officinale)

Licorice (Glycyrrhiza glabra)

Kava (Piper methysticum)

Yellow Dock (Rumex crispus)

Seeds or Berries

Elderberry (Sambucus nigra)

Fennel (Foeniculum vulgare)

Hawthorn (Crataegus species)

Milk Thistle (Silybum marianum)

Rose Hips (Rosa species)

Vitex (Vitex agnus-castus)

Bark

Cinnamon (Cinnamomum species)

Cramp Bark (Viburnum opulus)

Slippery Elm (Ulmus rubra)

Wild Cherry (Prunus serotina)

Willow (Salix alba)

Mushrooms

Chaga (Inonotus obliquus)

Cordyceps (Cordyceps sinensis)

Reishi (Ganoderma lucidum)

Recipes for Decoctions:

Blend for Detoxing

- 3 points- Milk Thistle

- 1 point- Gentian or Gentiana lutea

- 1.5 points- burdock (Arctium lappa).

- 1.5 points- Dandelion Root (Taraxacum officinale).

- 1 point for ginger (Zingiber officinale)

Adaptagen (to help the body deal with stress) Blend

- 4 points for Ashwagandha (Withania somnifera)

- 2 points: Eluthero (Elutherococcus senticosus)

- 0.5 points for licorice (Glycyrrhiza glabra)

How to make a hot Infusion

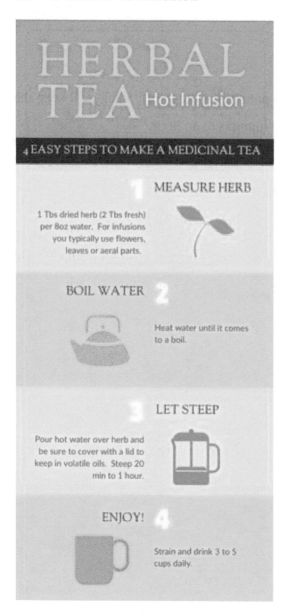

1. Measure the plant

2 tablespoon of fresh plant for every 8 ounces of water. Infusions usually have flowers, leaves, or parts of plants that grow above ground.

2. Heat Water Up

Bring water to a boil.

3. Let it steep.

Cover the flower with a lid and pour hot water over it. This will keep the volatile oils inside. Steep for 20 minutes to an hour.

Tip: Some herbs, like nettles, raspberry leaf, oatstraw, and red clover, are more helpful if you let them rest for longer.

4. Have fun!

You can strain it and drink it warm, or you can put it in the fridge or add ice to make it cold. You can also mix your tea with water, put it in a water bottle, and drink it all day. It could last up to a week if kept in the fridge.

Recipes for hot infusions:

Blend for Calming:

- 2 parts of Linden
- 1 part flower of love
- 1 part chamomile
- 1/2 of a rose petal
- 1/2 of a lavender
- A little bit of stevia leaf

How to Blend Something Cold:

1. Measure the plant

2 tablespoon of fresh plant for every 8 ounces of water. Most of the time, bitter herbs, mucilaginous herbs, and plants with delicate essential oils are

used for cold infusions. Some of these herbs are peppermint, marshmallow root, slippery elm, astragalus, licorice root, fresh lemon balm, fresh St. John's Wort, and fresh flowers like lavender and rose buds.

2. Let it steep.

Put a lid on top of the herb and pour cold water over it. Leave the injection alone for at least one hour, or even overnight.

How to Make a Cold Infusion:

Nosh Tamer Tea

- 2 pieces of marshmallow
- 1 part chamomile
- 1 part green
- ½ cup of fresh ginger

Tools for steeping tea:

- A French press makes it easy to make a lot of tea at once. It's great for brewing tea overnight, and the lid keeps the flammable oils inside.
- Another great choice is the Infuser Mug or Infuser Tea Pot. It has a lid that makes it easy to steep herbal tea the right way. When you're done steeping, you can use the cover as a tray for the filter.
- If you want to steep in a glass jar, you can strain with a tea ball, a muslin bag, or a bean screen.
- A cup top strainer is another good choice if you only want to make one cup of coffee. For this method, make sure you get a

mug with a lid or put something over the mug, like a plate, to let the tea simmer.

- A bombilla is a handy way to drink loose tea on the go. There's no need to push.

- You can take your tea with you anywhere with a tea mug. It can be used for hot or cold tea.

- You can strain the water through a cheesecloth if you want to put the herbs right into the water.

How much to use for infusions and decoctions:

- Please drink one cup of tea every two hours (while awake) if you have a short-term illness.

- Tea three to four times a day for people with long-term illnesses. Most of the time, we suggest using a restorative tea for a week or more.

- For kids, split the child's weight by 150 to get the right dose. A 75-pound child can have half of an adult dose, which is .5 times the adult amount.

- Dosage for babies: Twenty to thirty minutes after the mother drinks the tea, the babies can get the benefits of the medicine through breast milk. Just make sure that herbs are safe for you to eat while you are nursing.

It's both a science and an art to blend green tea. Do some study to find out which plants are safe to use with the medicines you are on, or work with a herbalist or naturopath to make a formula that is just right for you.

How to Make Herbal Lotions and Salve for the First Time

Putting herbal treatments on cuts, rashes, and dry, dull skin can be a nice way to help them feel better.

People often buy these at health food stores, but it's often quick and easy to make them at home. Topical treatments like these can not only feed your skin, but they can also help it absorb nutrients and protect it in a gentle way.

Creams, oils, and lotions

Herbal products that are put on the skin come in three main forms: infused oils, salves, and creams or lotions.

- **Infused** oils are made by letting herbs sit in a base oil like almond or olive oil for a while. This pulls out the healing parts of the plants that will help your skin.
- **Salves** are solid balms made of oils and a wax, like soy wax or beeswax.
- **Creams and lotions,** which you probably know, come in different thicknesses and consist of oils and water mixed together to make a moisturizing treatment for the skin.

Adding dried plants to oil is the first thing you need to do to make these remedies at home. If you want to treat the skin, you can use the oil by itself or mix it with other things to make a salve or cream.

You can mix and match oils for up to a year, so you can always have what you need in your home medicine kit.

Remember to do a patch test on your skin before putting anything new on it to avoid having an allergic reaction.

How to make an oil with herbs

This recipe makes about 8 ounces.

What you need:

- 4 oz. plant that has been dried
- 8 oz. olive oil, almond oil, or another oil that is good for the body
- mason jar that holds a quart
- stock pot or crock pot

What to do:

1. Add the dried plant to the mason jar after cutting it up or making a powder out of it. Cover with the oil and stir it in slowly to spread the herb out in the oil.
2. Put the lid on the mason jar and put it in a water bath in a crockpot or a stock pot on the stove. If you use a stock pot, put a mason jar lid ring under the jar with the oil in it so the glass doesn't touch the metal of the pot.
3. For three to five days, slowly heat the oil and water together, making sure the oil stays around 110 degrees. On a slow pot, the "warm" setting works best.
4. After 3–5 days, take the jar off the oil and let it cool down until it's not too hot to touch. Then, strain the oil to get rid of the dried herbs through cotton, cheesecloth, or an old, clean t-shirt.

5. Keep your oil in a dark, cool place in a jar that won't let air in. It has a year of use.

How to make a balm with herbs

This recipe makes about 9 ounces.

What you need:

- 8 oz. mixed with herbs oil
- 1 oz. beeswax, either small pieces or grated
- two boilers
- Clean metal or glass boxes
- essential oils, if you want them

What to do:

1. Warm up the oil in a double pot. Stir in the beeswax until it melts. You can see how thick your salve is by dipping a clean spoon into it and then freezing it for a few minutes. Feel free to add more beeswax if it's too soft.

2. Use old jam jars or small metal tins to store the salve while it is still warm. You only need a few drops of essential oils at this point. Add them and stir with a chopstick or another clean tool.

3. Put the lids on the jars and keep them somewhere dark and cool. The salve will last for a year.

How to make a cream with herbs

This recipe makes about 16 ounces.

What you need:

- 1 cup of rosewater or pure water

- 3/4 cup plant-based oil (almond or herb-infused oil)
- 1/2 oz.–1 oz. less beeswax for a lighter cream and more for a firmer one
- two boilers
- blender or hand-held blender
- Clean the jars made of glass
- essential oils, if you want them

What to do:

1. Put the beeswax and oil in a double pot and heat them slowly until the beeswax melts. Put the oil mix into a mixer, and then let it cool down to room temperature. The mix will get cloudy and build up.

2. Once it's cool, set the mixer to high speed and slowly pour a thin stream of water into the oil in the middle of the vortex. If your blender likes to get hot, you might need to stop and let it cool down before going on. The heat will melt the oil and beeswax again, which will stop the emulsion from working right.

3. Wait until the mixture goes white and gets thick to move on to the next step. As soon as the cream gets too stiff, the blender will start to stutter. It's okay if you don't use all the water.

4. Now is a good time to add essential oils. If you want to, fold in one or two drops slowly.

5. To get all of the cream out of the blender, use a spatula to pour it into the glass vessels. Put the lid on and keep it somewhere cool and dry. Creams can be kept for up to a month, and putting them in the fridge will make them last longer.

Bandage for cuts and scrapes

Note: Burns that are very bad need medical care. This cream works best on small cuts and burns. If you are worried, you should see a doctor.

What you need:

- 8 oz. herbal oil made from comfrey leaf (Symphytum sp.), oregon grape root (Berberis aquifolium), and calendula (Calendula officinalis) in equal amounts
- Between 1 and 2 drops of lavender oil

How to make rash cream

For a cool and healing experience, use aloe instead of some of the water in this cream.

What you need:

- 2/3 cup of distilled water
- 1/3 of a cup of aloe vera gel
- 3/4 cup of oil mixed with equal parts of marshmallow root (Althea officinalis), lemon balm (Melissa officinalis), and chamomile (Matricaria recutita).
- 1-2 drops of Melaleuca alternifolia tea tree oil

How to make radiant face cream

What you need:

- 1 cup of rose water
- 3/4 cups of oil mixed with yarrow (Achillea millefolium) and calendula (Calendula officinalis) in equal amounts.
- 1 to 2 drops of clary sage oil (Salvia sclarea)

What to Do

Now that you know how to make herbal remedies that you can put on your skin, you can try these easy recipes and fill your first-aid kit with natural remedies to help with cuts, rashes, dry patches, and other small injuries.

What You Should Know About Herbal Baths

Herbs are very useful. There are many ways we can cook them! Sheaves, teas, salves, powders, pills, sprays, compresses, poultices, steams, and herbal baths are just a few of the things we can do with them.

Everything You Need to Know About Herbal Baths

Taking a herb bath is a great way for anyone to enjoy the healing effects of herbs. Did you know that herbs can help with almost any illness when added to a bath? We all know how great it feels to sink into warm, healing water and feel joy bumps on your skin. A herbal bath is very helpful because it makes you feel good and contains healing qualities and active alkaloids that come from plants. One way to soak your whole body is in the tub. Another way is to make a small foot bath or a sitz bath for your bottom.

Pros of Taking Herbal Baths

Often, when we think of herbal treatments for the first time, we only picture herbal medicine in the form of pills, strange elixirs, or syrups. Remember that plant medicine is an old way of healing that comes from all over the world. It is not at all the same as prescription or over-the-counter drugs that contain chemicals. Instead, herbs are part of a healthy living and mending plan for the whole body.

The aromatic parts of the herbs we choose are mixed into the water when we take a bath with them. Herb baths are usually made up of herbs that reduce inflammation, kill germs, boost the immune system, calm the body, or help it heal itself.

The skin is the body's largest organ, so it's also a great way for the herbs' healing qualities to get into the body. Pathogens have a hard time getting into our bodies through our skin, which is also a strong defense.

The warm water opens up the pores, which helps the body stay hydrated and lets the herbs' benefits work their magic. When we work with plants, we also work with the natural ways that our bodies work. We need to soak in the water for at least 20 to 30 minutes for herb baths to work. This is important to know because your body is only hydrating for the first 15 minutes. The next 15 minutes are when the active herbal chemicals are absorbed. If you stay in for more than 30 minutes, you will start to lose water, so you won't get the full health benefits of plant baths.

Why Take A Bath With Herbs?

You can make a lot of different kinds of herb baths; it all depends on what you want to achieve. To help you focus on your goal, ask yourself: Why are you making a flower bath? Is it to help heal perineal tears, stitches, and body aches after giving birth? Do you want to make a drink with herbs because someone has a fever? For a cough, stuffy nose, and swollen lungs? Are you pregnant and sick with morning sickness and vomiting? Would you like to take a bath to help you stay hydrated? Are you trying to help your kid sleep better? Do you want to get rid of the pain and aches from cuts, bruises, and scrapes? Does your body only hurt and your head hurt?

Or do you want to clear your energy field and let go of negative feelings that you have been holding on to? Every one of these is a great reason to soak in herbs.

As you can see, plant baths are great for almost any reason. However, there are some situations where they work especially well, such as:

- **Postpartum-** healing after giving birth, pelvic floor healing, and body restoration
- **Babies**—to help dry out the umbilical cord, treat diaper rash and colic, and help parents bond
- **For kids**, it can help with bug bites, rashes, and growing pains during colds and flu.
- **For all ages,** it boosts the immune system and fights infections.
- **When it's cold and flu season**, it clears up stuffy noses, body aches, and fevers.
- **Clogged lungs**: gets rid of upper and lower respiratory illnesses
- **Detoxification**: getting rid of poisons that have been stored in the organs and skin
- **Relaxation**—relieves stress and strain in the body and mind
- **Sore muscles**: eases body aches and pains caused by stress or injury

- **For hemorrhoids**, it lowers swelling and heals damaged blood vessels and tissue.

- **Achy feet:** eases pain and wakes up tired, sore feet

- **To soak your hands** in warm water helps ease the pain of arthritis.

- **Take care of yourself**—do it with love and make it a goal.

Herbs that work best for herbal baths are:

How you answer the question "why make a herb bath?" will help you choose the best herbs for your bath. After you figure that out, it's easy to choose which plants to soak in.

For the most part, I use dried flower petals, leaves, or scents to make my baths. You can, of course, use fresh plants in your bath as well. I only use a few tried-and-true herbs that either increase blood flow, boost immunity, kill germs and keep infections away, help cells grow back, reduce inflammation, cleanse the body, or calm me down. Here are some of my favorites:

- Thyme is good for kids and kills germs, including strep.

- Lavender: calms you down and helps with pain and aches

- Yarrow is great for breastfeeding when you need strong first aid and immune-boosting.

- Calendula is good for your face, kills germs, and makes you happy.

- Peppermint: makes you feel good and wakes you up.

- Eucalyptus: clears up stuffy lungs and sinuses

- Plantain is good for healing wounds and bruises and making skin feel better.

- Ceremonial sage gets rid of negative feelings and blocks.

- Dandelion: cleans the body

When you are choosing herbs and making your mix, keep in mind that mood and pleasure can heal. For instance, some flowers may be very soothing and good for pain and stress, but they smell awful. This is shown very clearly by Valerian. Either don't use it or mix small amounts of it with herbs that smell better. Just make sure you know what the smell is like before you soak your plants.

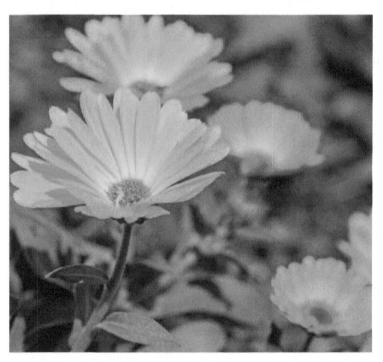

When to make herbal baths and how to do it:

You can make a herb bath in a full soaking tub, a sitz bath, or a foot bath with less herbs. Think about what you want to get out of the bath and whether you need to soak only a small part of your body or your whole body.

Make a strong "tea" from a cup or two of dried herbs for a full bath to make a herb bath. You could also put salts in it. When you use essential oils, pick oils that are mild and mix them with salts first, since oil and water don't mix. The salts will help them spread out more evenly.

To make the bath stronger, put the herbs in a cheesecloth or pantyhose sock satchel and tie it up. Then, put the satchel right into the water. You can get even more health benefits from the herbs by massaging the bundle while you're in the bath.

Really, I hope you can see how simple it is to make a herb bath and how important it is to use simple things to treat many problems. Herbs, water, and heat.

Chapter 5

Specialized Herbal Treatments

Herbs For Immune Stimulants, Immunomodulators, and Antimicrobials

We'll start with ways of living that are good for your immune system before we talk about herbs. It's because herbs are the cherry on top of the cake, while the decisions we make every day about how we want to live are the cake. Things in life that make us feel healthy, happy, linked, and full of energy also make our immune cells feel strong and alert. Our feelings are very important to how our immune systems work. In fact, psychoneuroimmunology is a whole field of study about this. The way we feel and our feelings have a big impact on our white blood cells, which are immune cells like B cells, T cells, natural killer (NK) cells, and macrophages. The biggest "downers" on the immune system are worry and being alone. Stress chemicals like cortisol and adrenaline (epinephrine) make the immune system less strong. On the other hand, when we are happy and relaxed, our cells make neural signaling molecules like serotonin, dopamine, and relaxin, which make our immune systems stronger.

420 people took part in a study that was published in the New England Journal of Medicine. They chose to snort either a nose spray solution that contained the cold virus or a placebo. The volunteers who said they were very stressed before being exposed were more likely to get a cold, while those who said they were less stressed were more likely to be able to fight off the virus.1 Stress can also change how our immune cells deal with

69

cancerous cells. At least two studies have shown that helping cancer patients deal with worry can raise immune factors that can be measured. In a study with melanoma cancer patients, one group learned how to relax for six weeks, while the control group did not learn any ways to deal with worry. Natural killer cells (NK cells) were much more active in the rest group than in the control group.2 NK cells are white blood cells that are always looking for cancerous cells in the body and killing them. They are often used to measure how resistant people are to cancer because they are so important to the body's defense against it. In a similar study, people with breast cancer who took a ten-week course on stress management were compared to people who did not take the training. At the end of the program, people who took the stress management course had higher numbers of white blood cells than people in the control group.3

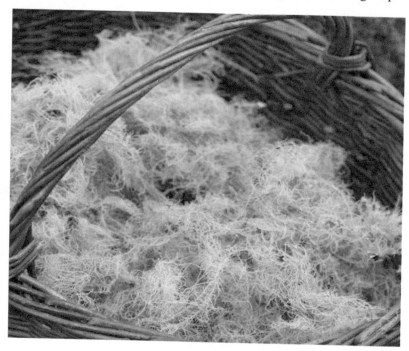

Lichen of Usnea

As everyone knows, people are social animals who need each other to survive and feel better. Sadly, the society of modern industrialized countries, especially the US, downplays interdependence and instead praises extreme independence and a false sense of being able to do everything on your own. It's more important for health and immunity than you might think to feel linked and like someone "has our back." One big study of breast cancer survivors found that women who didn't have many friends were four times more likely to die of cancer than women who did have a lot of friends.4 Being lonely is linked to higher cortisol levels and a weaker immune system.5 Our human bonds don't have to be family; we can find community and friendship through our hobbies, work, support groups, volunteering, church, or spiritual groups.

It's likely already clear to you that sleep and defense are linked. People who have been busy for a long time know that not getting enough sleep is one of the fastest ways to get a cold.

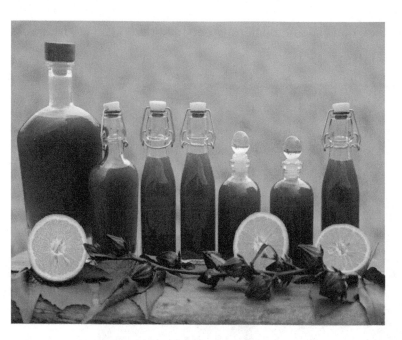

Fire Cider with Hibiscus, Pomegranate, and Orange

Nutrition is also very important for defense. To keep your immune system strong, you need to get enough zinc, vitamins D and C. Bell pepper, broccoli, Brussels sprouts, papaya, oranges, strawberries, and pineapple are all good sources of vitamin C.6 Oysters, beef, crab, and lobster are all high in zinc, but chicken, cheese, kidney beans, garbanzo beans, cashews, and almonds are not as high.

Lastly, it's important for making vitamin D to spend time in the sun during the middle of the day with your skin uncovered. People with darker skin or who live far from the equator are more likely to not get enough vitamin D. It's not as easy to find vitamin D and food sources. Some of these foods are wild salmon, sardines, fish liver oil, mushrooms that have been dried out in the sun, and to a lesser extent, cow's milk and eggs.8 Many people choose to take vitamin D supplements to make sure they get enough, especially if they don't spend much time outside or are in an at-risk group as described above.

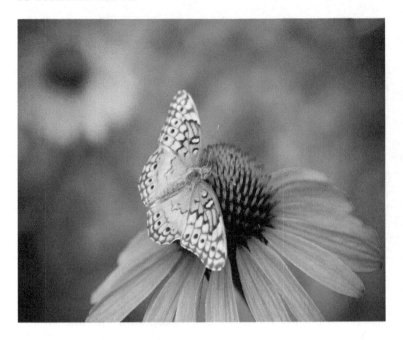

Purple Echinacea

Wendell Berry does a great job of summing up a whole-person approach to healing in The Unsettling of America:

"Our bodies are not separate from the bodies of plants and animals. We are connected to them in the cycles of feeding and in the complex relationships of the spirit and ecological systems." They are the same as the earth, the sun, the moon, and all the other celestial things. So, it makes no sense to approach the subject of health in pieces with a group of specialists from different departments. A doctor who doesn't care about nutrition, farming, or the health of the mind and spirit is just as silly as a farmer who doesn't care about health. The way we've broken up this subject can't be our cure; it's our illness.

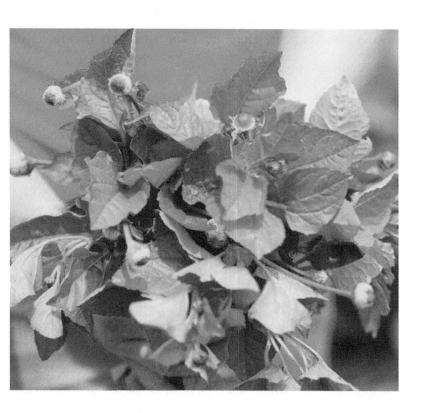

Spilanthes plant (Acmella oleracea)

It's important to know that herbs aren't always the only thing you need to fight infections, especially if the infections are very dangerous or contagious. Trust your own judgment and gut feelings, and learn to spot the signs of conditions that could be very dangerous. Improve your faith and wisdom so you can know when to go to a regular doctor. It's better to be safe than sorry, and herbal ideals shouldn't get in the way of getting better. Parents and other adults who care for children: you are their best friend and biggest supporter. Talk up if your doctor or other health care worker does or says something that doesn't seem right. You know important things about your child's health that can help your doctor make a choice or make a diagnosis. Here are some situations in which you should go to a regular doctor.

When to Ask for Help

If you have any of these possibly dangerous symptoms, please call your doctor or go to the emergency room right away:

- Feeling very tired, with or without a fever. If your child doesn't want to play or eat at all and just seems really "off," you should call the doctor.
- A baby younger than three months can have a fever of more than 100.4°F (38°C).
- A fever of more than 103.5°F (39.7°C) or a fever that lasts for more than three days.
- Rapid, short breathing and wheezing sounds when you try to breathe.
- An earache, sore throat, strong headache, or stomachache that won't go away or is very painful...
- A red line coming from a cut.
- Vomiting or diarrhea a lot: If your child hasn't gone to the bathroom in eight to twelve hours, they may be dehydrated. Lack of tears when crying, dry lips, a soft fontanel (a soft spot on a baby's skull), and sunken eyes are some other signs of dehydration. There should also be no blood in the vomit or feces.
- Headaches, fever, and a stiff neck are all signs that you might have meningitis. Most of the time, a child with meningitis only

shows two of the three symptoms mentioned above. A bulging fontanel (soft spot) in a baby's head can be a sign of meningitis or other possibly serious conditions. When a baby is crying, sitting down, or throwing up, the fontanels may swell. When the baby is calm and standing up, the fontanels should return to normal. If an infant has a bulging fontanel and is also tired or feverish, they need medical care right away.

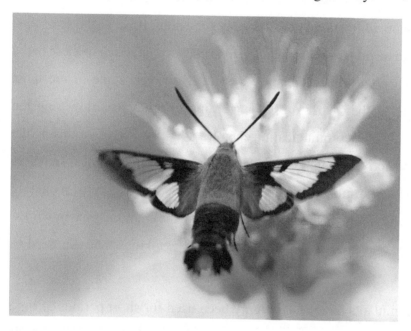

Wild bergamot (Monarda fistulosa) flowers are a food source for the clearwing hummingbird moth.

Immunostimulants from plants

Short-term use of this group of plants is used to treat acute infections by making white blood cells work harder. In addition to being called immune boosters, immunoostimulants help the body fight off infections both before they happen and while they are happening. You can also use herbs that boost the immune system when you are around someone who has a contagious disease. Take Spilanthes with me whenever I fly to help my body deal with the higher quantity and wider range of pathogens in the cabin air. Many of the following herbs are also antimicrobial, which means they work double duty by both boosting the body's defense system and killing the pathogen directly.

These plants, which are also known as surface immune activators, work right away on white blood cells but only for a short time. Because of this, they need to be given again and again to keep working. Each of these herbs has its own effect on the defense system. However, some of the most common ways they work are by increasing phagocytosis, lowering the amount of defense communication chemicals like cytokines, or raising the number and activity of white blood cells. Cytokines are chemical signalers that work like hormones and are made by many types of cells, including immune cells. They have big impacts on how the immune system works. Interleukins and interferons are two types of cytokines that you need to know about.

Immunostimulants have usually only been used for short periods of time because they are very exciting and can throw your body out of balance if you use them for a long time. Many of them heat up and spread out, which can be uncomfortable for people with hot bodies (like those who run hot, are often short-tempered or emotional, and are prone to inflammation). It's possible for immunosuppressants to make autoimmunity worse, and while this doesn't happen very often, it has happened to people with autoimmune diseases.

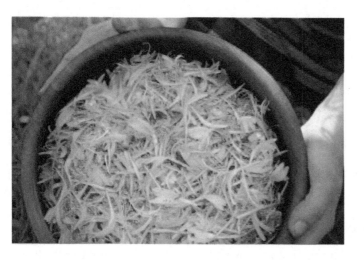

Lonicera japonica, or Japanese honeysuckle

This needs to be said again because it's too easy to "prop ourselves up" with immune boosters while we ignore taking care of our body, feelings, and spirit. When someone dies from an infectious disease, it's important to look at the body's state, or "terrain," and figure out how the infection got there. To get the most out of antibacterial and immune-stimulating herbs, we should not forget about the basics like getting enough sleep, eating well, drinking water, and living a healthy lifestyle. It's not a complete way to heal to treat symptoms without changing the unhealthy things that are happening. The American Herbal Pharmacopoeia recently tested forty samples of botanically-verified boneset and found that it has low amounts of pyrrolizidine alkaloids (PAs), especially intermedine and lycopsamine, which can be harmful. Until more research is done, we advise women who are pregnant or nursing not to use boneset internally. Also, people who are known to have liver disease or are younger than 12 years old should not take it by mouth. Others who want to take boneset by mouth (after learning about the possible liver damage caused by PA) should not do so for more than one week and should ideally take the herb in a mixture with other herbs to lower the dose.

August 2021: A safety update: Boneset has pyrrolizidine alkaloids (PAs) in it, which can hurt the liver over time if taken by mouth. The PAs in boneset and other plants that contain them can be taken up by other plants when they are grown close to each other or when comfrey is used as mulch or fertilizer in the yard. Since this is the case, we suggest that boneset not be put near herbs or food plants that will be eaten or that will be used as mulch or fertilizer. This is just to be safe. However, PAs don't seem to be in adult compost that has boneset in it after it has been fully composted.

Immunomodulators from plants

These plants have been used for a long time to support the immune system. They work more slowly than immunostimulants but for a longer time. They are used for longer amounts of time and have a more balancing effect on the body than a stimulating one. They are also known as deep immune tonics or immune amphoterics. As tonics, they don't overly warm or stimulate, and they work well for a lot of different types of constitutions. Look at how each herb has been used traditionally and how it affects the body to find the solution that works best for each person.

These herbs are used in medicine to help people whose immune systems aren't strong enough, like those who get sick a lot. Herbal immunomodulators are also used when the immune system is working too hard, like in asthma and autoimmunity. This nature that seems to have two sides can seem impossible at first, especially to people who know how drugs work in only one way. First, think about the fact that most plants have thousands of bioactive compounds. The biochemistry of each herb is very complicated, but they all work together very well. When we take into account that every person's body is different, the results that could happen are almost endless. Also, as we'll talk about in more depth below, immunomodulators help the nervous and endocrine systems work together properly, which in turn controls immunity.

A lot of immunomodulators are also adaptogens. Adaptogens are tonic herbs that help the body deal with physical, mental, and emotional stress. Some of the magic that herbal immunomodulators do is by balancing the immune system's control by the senses and the brain. These tonic plants help to balance the hypothalamic-pituitary-adrenal axis, which affects how hormones control the immune system. This makes the body's control centers work better. The balance of T helper cells (Th1 and Th2) is another way it might work. This includes the balance of cell-mediated (T cells) and antibody-mediated (B cells) defense.

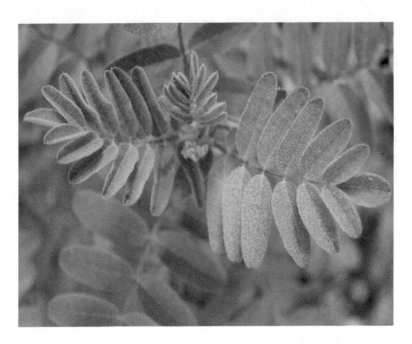

That's Astragalus membranaceus.

If you want to boost your immune system and lower your risk of getting common viruses in the fall and winter, you can take herbal immunomodulators every day. This group of herbs can also help avoid and treat cancer. Many of them are adaptogens that are used along with standard cancer treatments like chemotherapy and radiation. To stop cancer, you might want to look into immunomodulators that work as antioxidants and lower the body's general inflammatory nature. This lowers the ability of free radicals to cause mutations and the role of inflammation in the progression of cancer.

In a slightly different setting, the word "immunomodulation" can also be used for drugs. It is predictable that pharmaceutical immunomodulators will either boost or weaken the immune system at their target site, but their effects rely on the target site. People with cancer are given them to boost their immune systems, while people with autoimmunity and graft or organ donations are given them to weaken them.

Keep in mind that a lot of the herbs on this list are from Asia. This is just because people and governments in Asian countries are interested in herbal drugs and fund research into them. Most of these medicines can be grown in a home garden, and many of them are already being grown on a big scale in people's yards. Many Western herbs that are used to boost the immune system are also likely to be immunomodulators, even if they don't have the official "stamp of approval" for that.

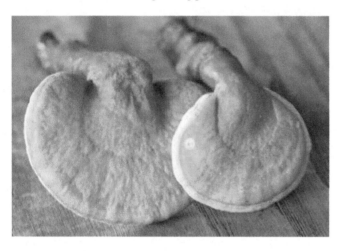

Ganoderma lucidum, or Reishi

Herbal Immune Spikes

These herbs have been used for a long time to boost the immune system, and they probably also have affects that change the immune system. They can be used for a long time to treat and avoid cancer, as well as people who don't have a strong immune system. Perhaps you want to know what the difference is between an immunomodulator and an immunity tonic. Most of the time, herbal immunity tonics and herbal immunomodulators are used in the same way. There isn't enough scientific proof for immune tonics to be called immunomodulators, but they may have similar effects on controlling or balancing the immune system.

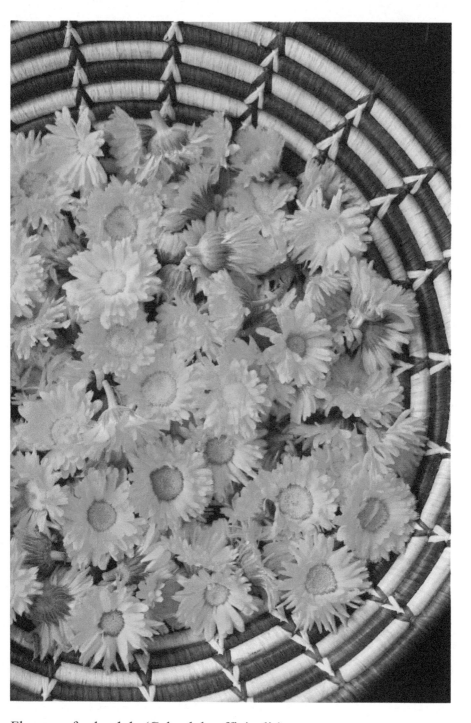

Flowers of calendula (Calendula officinalis)

84

Herbal Antimicrobial

Herbs that are antimicrobial have chemicals in them that directly kill harmful bacteria, fungi, viruses, and protozoans. These leaves can be used in a lot of different ways. A lot of these plants are effective against more than one type of pathogen. One plant might be able to kill both bacteria and protozoa, while another might be able to kill both viruses and bacteria. If you want to use herbs to treat an illness, it helps to know what kind of infection you have and how well those herbs work against that infection.

It's interesting to know that most traditional cooking herbs have strong antimicrobial properties that keep food from going bad and stop enteric pathogens from spreading. I can say for sure that raw garlic, cayenne, and oregano keep food fresh because I lived in a subtropical environment for years without being able to cool my food. From my own experience, dishes that weren't spiced went bad days faster than foods that were spiced a lot.

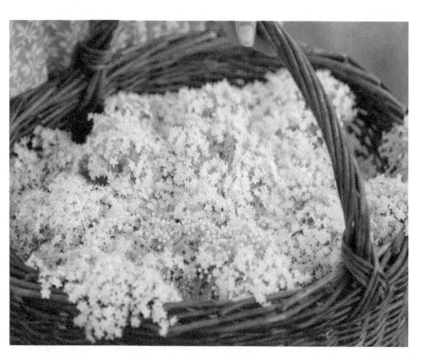

The elderflower harvest

Antibiotics, antifungals, antiprotozoans, and other related drugs have saved a huge number of lives when it comes to fighting infectious organisms. There is no doubt that these remedies work, but they need to be taken in the right way or they can have side effects like fewer good bacteria and bacteria that are immune to antibiotics. Herbal antimicrobial treatments can help with the common cold, the flu, and other light to moderate infections that are easy to handle.

Natural Pain Relievers

You can get pain relief in more ways than just by taking painkillers. If you have a toothache, back pain, or any other kind of pain, you can try turmeric, which is a natural plant that can help.

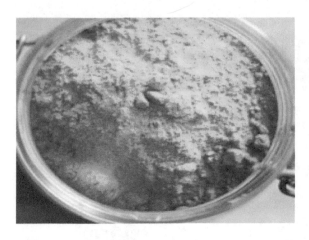

Natural ways to ease pain

If you're in pain, like from a toothache, backache, or something else, you might want to take a painkiller right away.

A lot of people depend on medications, but there is a chance that they will have side effects, combine with other drugs, or be abused.

There are times when you may need a prescription or over-the-counter (OTC) pain medicine, but there are also natural pain relievers that may help you feel better. A lot of plants and spices have been used for a long time to ease pain and inflammation.

These natural pain killers are part of a type of care called "alternative medicine," which also includes acupuncture, yoga, reiki, and other methods.

There are some good things about using natural treatments to ease pain and inflammation, but keep in mind that they can sometimes interact badly with other medicines you are taking.

Also, some natural pain killers haven't been studied well enough in people (especially when it comes to dosage), and a lot of supplements aren't tested by a third-party lab to make sure they're safe or of good quality. In the same way that drugs are controlled by the Food and Drug Administration (FDA), supplements are not.

It's best to talk to a doctor before getting any natural remedies if you're in pain or have long-term problems. Integrative medicine doctors, who are doctors who have training in more natural treatments, may be a good choice if you're looking for different ways to treat pain.

A qualified health worker should also be consulted before adding any supplements to your routine. This is especially important if you already have a health problem or are taking other medicines.

Boswellia

Linalool, which is another name for boswellia, is often used in Ayurvedic medicine. Boswellia serrata tree resin is often used to make tinctures, pills, or products that you put on your skin.

What does it treat?

A lot of people use boswellia to:

- signs of asthma
- joint pain
- colitis (an swollen gut)
- inflammation in general
- lessening of cerebral edema (swelling of the brain caused by fluid)
- Less damage to the skin from radiotherapy

A 2020 study with 545 people found that Boswellia was a safe and effective way to treat osteoarthritis (OA), making pain and stiffness less severe.

Effects that could happen

Boswellia is usually safe, but some people can have an allergic response to it when they put it on their skin. It may also have bad effects when mixed with some medicines, like blood thinners and clotting drugs.

If you are taking one of these medicines, Boswellia extract may make you more likely to bleed.

Turmeric

Curry has a unique yellow color and taste that come from the spice turmeric.

It has an antioxidant in it called curcumin that helps keep the body safe from free radicals that can hurt cells. A lot of research has also been done on how well it can ease swelling and reduce inflammation.

Turmeric is usually used as a spice, but it can also be bought as a vitamin, and it is often mixed with piperine, a chemical found in black pepper, to help the body absorb it better.

What does it treat?

Turmeric might help with a lot of different health problems, such as:

- stomach pain
- sores
- upset stomach
- eczema`

- swelling brought on by conditions like OA

Effects that could happen

Turmeric is usually thought to be safe, but some people have experienced some negative effects.

Here are some of the most common side effects:

- sickness
- belly pain
- migraines
- hives
- a yellow poop

Before taking turmeric pills, you should talk to a doctor. If you experience any bad affects, stop using them.

Cloves

To make pork and rice taste better, whole cloves are often added. Cloves that have been ground are used in pies and many other foods.

Eugenol, which is found in cloves and is also used in some over-the-counter pain rubs, is a natural pain relief that is often used to treat pain.

You can get cloves in the form of capsules or powder. You can also get clove oil, which can be put on the skin to ease pain.

What does it treat?

You can use clove to treat a lot of different things, like

- sickness
- getting colds

- migraines
- inflammation from arthritis
- sore teeth
- stomach pain
- belly pain

Some studies also show that clove might be able to help with fungal diseases, but we need more high-quality studies on people.

Effects that could happen

When cloves are taken as a supplement, they might cause side affects like

- problems with the liver
- response to allergies
- irritation of skin
- more blood loss

Clove oil can be put on the skin to help with things like toothache pain, but if you don't dilute it first, it could hurt your gums, so talk to your doctor before you try it at home.

People who have problems with bleeding or who take medicines that thin the blood should also be careful when eating clove goods because clove and clove oil can make bleeding more likely.

Because of this, you should talk to a doctor before taking herbal products with clove in them.

Acupuncture

This old Chinese medicine method tries to ease pain by restoring balance to the body's energy pathways. Qi (pronounced "chee") is the flow of energy.

Tiny, thin needles are put into your skin by acupuncturists for this treatment. The source of the pain is linked to where the injection is. Based on the qi, the needle may be put in a place other than the painful area of the body.

The body may release serotonin, a "feel-good" chemical that eases pain, when you get acupuncture. Some people also think it can lower stress and help the body heal.

What does it treat?

Acupuncture may help with a number of different kinds of pain, such as:

- OA in the knee
- headache
- pain in the muscles
- short-term and long-term low back pain
- low back pain
- pain in the neck

Effects that could happen

Acupuncture may be linked to a number of possible side effects.

Here are some of the most common side effects:

- damage to an organ, tissue, or nerve
- skin problems
- response to allergies

- more blood loss
- losing consciousness

Before you try acupuncture, you should talk to your doctor to make sure it's safe for you.

- have a heart pacemaker
- you are pregnant
- have problems with bleeding
- take medicines that thin the blood, like warfarin

Ice and heat

Putting heat and ice directly on painful areas is one of the most popular ways to treat pain at home. Even though this technique may seem clear, not everyone knows when to use heat and when to use ice.

If you have a pulled muscle, tendon, or ligament, putting an ice pack on it right away may help reduce swelling and pain.

It's interesting that heat may help ease the stiffness that comes with sprains and strains after the swelling goes down.

A heating pad or cold pack put on the head for a short time may also help ease the pain of a headache. An ice pack, on the other hand, can help ease the pain of low back pain.

People with arthritis will feel better when they apply wet heat to the painful joint instead of ice. You can warm up moist heat packs in the microwave and use them more than once. This makes them useful and simple to use.

What does it treat?

The use of an ice pack may help with problems such as

- swell-up
- being bleed
- pain or swelling
- migraines
- back pain
- muscles, tendons, or ligaments that are strained

On the other hand, using heat can help with situations like:

- a stiff joint
- spasms of muscles
- joint pain
- migraines

Effects that could happen

If you put heat or ice on an injury for too long, you might get burns or other problems.

These are some of the most common side effects of heat or cold therapy:

- gets burned
- cuts or burns from ice
- feeling numb
- itchy skin
- pain
- sore feet

Talk to your doctor or pharmacist about how to use heat or ice to help ease pain if you get hurt or have long-term pain.

Be careful how you deal with pain.

It's possible that the natural pain killers we talked about above will only help with certain kinds of pain and won't help everyone.

But these natural choices might give you a few things to try, either by themselves or along with over-the-counter or prescription drugs.

Pain is your body's way of telling you that something is wrong. It could be short-term, like when you strain a muscle, or it could be a sign of a major health problem that needs medical help.

Please don't be afraid to see a doctor to find out what's causing your pain and talk about the best ways to treat it.

Also, you should always talk to your doctor or pharmacist before taking any herbal products or vitamins, especially if you already have a health problem or are taking other medicines.

Herbs that can help with arthritis pain

Different kinds of arthritis can cause pain that might not go away even after standard treatments. If you use natural remedies along with other treatments, they may help you deal with mild problems.

Some herbs can help with the pain of rheumatoid arthritis (RA) or osteoarthritis (OA) because they reduce inflammation.

Still, scientists need more proof to back their use and learn more about the bad effects they might have.

Before using herbs to treat gout, you should talk to a doctor. Some choices may not work well with medicines you are already taking.

1. **Aloe vera**

In alternative treatment, aloe vera is often used. It comes in a lot of different forms, like

- tablets
- flour
- gel
- leaf

Aloe vera is often used to treat small cuts and scrapes on the skin, like sunburn. It may also help with joint pain.

Some possible perks are:

- has traits that reduce inflammation
- can usually be handled well
- doesn't have the stomach problems that nonsteroidal anti-inflammatory drugs (NSAIDs), which are often used to treat joint pain, do

A gel can be put on the skin immediately. In 2014, some experts said that taking aloe by mouth might help ease the pain of OA.

To be sure that these treatments work, more research needs to be done.

The National Center for Complementary and Integrative Health (NCCIH) says that using aloe vera is probably safe, but taking it by mouth may make some people feel bad.

It might lower glucose levels and change how some diabetes medicines work.

2. **Boswellia**

Boswellia serrata, which is also known as frankincense, can help reduce inflammation and is used in both traditional and alternative treatment. Boswellia trees, which are native to India, are used to make one.

Some research from 2019 says that boswellic acid might help people with RA, bronchial asthma, ulcerative colitis, and other inflammatory diseases by reducing inflammation.

Studies with real people have shown that frankincense pills may help ease the pain, stiffness, and loss of function caused by OA. But these studies were not very big. We need to do more study.

Up to 1 gram of boswellia a day seems to be safe, but large amounts can hurt the liver. It comes in pill form and as a cream that you put on your skin.

3. A cat's claw

One more herb that may help lower swelling in arthritis is cat's claw. It comes from the root and bark of a tropical plant that grows in Central and South America.

In the past, people have used it to reduce inflammation and make their immune systems stronger.

A group called the Arthritis Foundation says that cat's claw, like many common drugs for RA, blocks tumor necrosis factor.

They talk about a small study from 2002 that showed cat's claw could help 40 people with RA reduce joint swelling by more than 50%.

However, some possible side affects are:

- feeling sick and dizzy

- not enough blood flow
- a headache

If these things are true, don't use this herb:

- take medicines that thin the blood
- take medicines that weaken the immune system
- you have tuberculosis

The NCCIH says that cat's claw has been looked at for RA in a few small studies, but more research is needed.

4. Eucalyptus

Eucalyptus is easy to get and is used to treat a lot of different problems. Extracts of eucalyptus leaves are used to treat arthritis pain on the skin.

Tannins, which are found in the plant's leaves, may help reduce joint pain and swelling. Some people use heat pads afterward to get the most out of the experience.

Essential oils of eucalyptus may help ease the pain of RA.

Before you use an essential oil, you should always mix it with a carrier oil. It's best to mix 15 drops of oil with 2 cups of almond oil or another neutral oil.

Before you use medicinal eucalyptus, you should do a patch test to see if you are allergic to it. Just put a little of the item on your hand. If there is no response in 24 to 48 hours, it should be safe.

5. Ginger

Ginger is often used in food, but it may also be good for you in other ways. According to study from 2016, the compounds that give ginger its strong flavor can also help reduce inflammation.

Some experts think ginger could one day be used instead of NSAIDs.

Ginger has been used for a long time to help people who feel sick. It can also help with RA, OA, and joint and muscle pain.

Researchers who wrote an older review of study from 2014 think that some of the ingredients in ginger could one day be used to make a drug that treats rheumatoid arthritis. It might not only help with symptoms, but it might also stop bones from breaking down.

There are different ways to eat ginger. Some of these are:

- Making tea by letting fresh ginger or tea bags steep in hot water for 5 minutes
- putting ginger powder in baked goods
- Making savory recipes with ginger powder or fresh ginger root
- putting grated fresh ginger on a stir-fry or salad

It's not clear if the high quantity of active ingredients in ginger tea will help ease symptoms. When ginger is eaten or drunk, it may not contain as much of it as when it is taken as a supplement.

You can talk to your doctor about taking ginger supplements and how much you should take to feel the effects.

Before you eat more ginger, talk to your doctor because it can interact with some drugs, like the blood thinner warfarin (Coumadin).

How to take ginger off

What to Do to Peel Ginger

It's Ginger

6. Green Tea

Many people like to drink green tea. It might help fight the inflammation that comes with RA or OA because it has vitamins in it.

Green tea can be drunk in the following ways:

- a drink
- matcha powder that can be used to sprinkle on food or mix into drinks
- extra foods

Scientists have found evidence that some parts or extracts of green tea may have an effect on arthritis. However, it's not clear if the amount of active ingredients in a cup of green tea will help reduce symptoms.

Still, most people should be fine with it. If you don't add sugar, it might be better for you than some coffees, sodas, and other sugary drinks as a drink.

More study is needed to prove that green tea can help reduce inflammation and figure out the best way to drink it and how much to drink.

7. Thunder god vine

The plant known as thunder god vine (Tripterygium wilfordii) is a vegetable. In Chinese, Japanese, and Korean medicine, it has been used for a long time to treat inflammation and overactive immune systems.

Because of this, it might be a good way to treat RA and other autoimmune illnesses.

It can be used for:

- by mouth as an addition to a healthy diet
- as a treatment that is put on the skin directly

It can, however, have very bad results, such as

- problems with the stomach
- infections of the lungs
- losing hair
- a headache
- a rash on the skin
- changes in your period
- changes in sperm that could make men less fertile
- After five years or more of use, it may make bones less dense

Thunder god vine can interact with a lot of medicines, especially those used to treat RA and other autoimmune illnesses.

Getting the extract from the wrong part of the plant can be dangerous. It's also important to keep in mind that the Food and Drug Administration (FDA) doesn't control the making or selling of herbal medicines.

You can't always be sure of what's in a product, and thunder god vine herb can be dangerous if it's not made right.

The NCCIH says there isn't enough proof to show that thunder god vine is safe or works to treat arthritis.

If used while pregnant, it could cause birth problems.

You should talk to a doctor about this herb. There may be other treatments that work better and have lower risks.

You shouldn't take thunder god vine over the counter. Someone who is qualified to prescribe herbal medicine might be able to give you a dose or formula that includes this herb.

8. Turmeric

The flower of the turmeric plant is used to make the yellow powder. It makes sweet and savory foods and drinks taste better and look better.

Curcumin, which is its main ingredient, can help reduce inflammation. It has been used in Ayurvedic and Chinese healing for a long time. It might help people with OA, RA, and other types of arthritis.

You can get turmeric:

- as a spice powder to put on food
- in bags of tea
- in pill form to be taken by mouth

There needs to be more research on how safe and useful turmeric is. The NCCIH says it's probably safe for most people, but some may have stomach problems if they take large amounts or use it for a long time.

People who practice Ayurvedic or Chinese medicine may give you turmeric as part of a mixture with other ingredients. A trained and approved herbal medicine practitioner might be able to give you a formula that includes turmeric.

9. Bark from willows

A review of the study done in 2015 says that willow bark extract has been used for thousands of years to ease pain, reduce swelling, and lower fevers.

Willow bark can be made into tea or tablets.

Some older study from 2009 suggests that it may help ease the pain of OA and RA joints. But the effects have been mixed, and more research is needed. It might not be safe for everyone either.

Some common side effects are:

- upset stomach
- a high heart rate
- an allergic reaction, this is especially true if you are allergic to aspirin
- stomach sores and bleeding if you take too much

Do not use willow bark until you talk to your doctor, especially if you are taking blood thinners or have a stomach infection. Should not be taken by people who are allergic to aspirin.

Salicin, which is found in white willow bark, is the chemical that scientists used to make aspirin.

Other choices that go well with

Herbal pills aren't the only way to help relieve the pain of arthritis.

The American College of Rheumatology and the Arthritis Foundation both have experts who say the following:

- controlling your weight
- exercise, like yoga and tai chi
- Care with cold and heat
- Dealing with fear
- A healthy meal plan
- pain relief

A study done in 2021 found that acupuncture helped people with OA feel less pain and do more.

Can what you eat help treat osteoarthritis? Read this to find out.

A doctor can tell you about alternative medicine.

Doctors who don't use herbal medicine are more ready to look into the benefits of alternative treatments as interest in them grows.

Some herbs may help your present arthritis medicines work better. But it's important to know that herbs can have very bad affects.

It's also important to make sure you get herbal remedies from a trustworthy source.

Since the FDA doesn't check herbs for quality, purity, packing, or dosage, you can't be sure if a product is tainted or has inactive ingredients.

A few supplement companies may pay for tests to be done by someone else.

Talk to your doctor about all of your arthritis treatment choices, and don't stop taking your medications unless they tell you to. You should never stop taking a medicine your doctor has recommended without their permission. To avoid major side effects, some medicines need to be slowly lowered in dose.

The American Association of Neuropathic Physicians may be able to help you find a licensed doctor who can recommend herbal medicine.

What to Do

Herbal cures may help ease the pain and swelling that come with RA, especially if they are used along with standard treatments.

Some qualified medical professionals may suggest supplements, exercise, acupuncture, and other non-drug treatments to help ease the symptoms of RA.

Herbal Medicine For Well Women Care

These days, most women in developed countries use allopathic medicine and drugs to treat and keep their reproductive health in check. Conventional medicine is important and has its place, but nature often has better ways to treat problems that are better for everyone.

An important part of most, if not all, traditional types of medicine is using herbs. It is based on the idea that people are connected to nature and that the solutions to our problems are often right outside our doors. Plants can help our bodies fix themselves and give us more control over them than other types of medicine. They may even be easier to get to than other types of medicine.

It might seem hard at first to learn how to use herbs to treat women's health problems, especially if you've never done it before. But trust your gut. You might have to wait a while before you find what works for you, but there are many tried-and-true solutions that have been shown to work many times.

Learning about the different ways you can eat herbs is important before learning about which herbs may be good for you.

- **Tea:** This is something we all know. A lot of people don't know this, but this practice is an important part of herbalism. A gentle way to start learning about herbs is to make tea from fresh or dried herbs that have already been mixed or that you have made yourself.

- **Tinctures:** These are concentrated plant extracts that are usually kept fresh in alcohol.

- **Capsules:** Herbs that are ground up and put into tiny gel pills are called capsules. You can even use a capsule kit to make your own.

- **Important Oils:** Essential oils are becoming more and more famous, and many people keep them in their home apothecaries. If you mix clary sage, ylang, ylang, and lavender with a carrier oil and rub it on your stomach, it can help ease menstrual cramps.

- **Salve:** As well as their healing properties, herbs are often added to many cosmetic treatments to make them smell nice.

Now that we know how, let's talk about what. In the world of natural medicine for women, these herbs are often used.

- **Black cohosh:** This herb can help with both menstrual cramps and hot flashes during menopause.

- **Calendula**, which is also called marigold, is known for its ability to reduce swelling and help wounds heal. Calendula cleans the body and makes the defense system stronger. In addition, it can help ease sore breasts and cramps.

- **Chamomile buds:** This happy bud is well known for its ability to calm people down. By easing blood vessels, glycine in chamomile helps ease muscle contractions, also known as cramps.

- **The Dong Quai:** is a Chinese medicine power play. It is thought to help women deal with the signs of menopause and PMS by making their hormones more flexible.
- **Fennel seeds:** Fennel is often used to treat gas, bloating, and stomach problems. It can also help with period pains.
- **Hibiscus:** Hibiscus protects the liver with its vitamins and nutrients, and the flavonoids in it can help calm the nervous system, which can make you feel better. Increasing blood flow to your pelvic area can also help keep your cycle in check.
- **Lady's Mantle:** This plant calms PMS symptoms and can even lighten a heavy flow. It also helps keep your cycle regular.
- **Nettles:** This stinging "weed" is high in minerals and can be found growing wild in many places. It has a lot of health benefits, like cleaning the liver and kidneys of toxins and helping people with anemia because it has a lot of iron.
- **Oat Straw:** Oatstraw is safe to take at any time during the reproductive cycle, even while breastfeeding or pregnant. It calms the body and removes stress.
- **Red Raspberry Leaf:** This herb can help with PMS signs like cramps and loose stools. People know that it can tone and strengthen the uterus, which can help with heavy or unpredictable periods, cramps, and even labor. This is mostly because it has a lot of calcium and magnesium in it. Not getting enough minerals is a big reason why women get period pains.
- **Rose buds:** In traditional Chinese medicine, beautiful rose buds are often used to help women with menstrual cramps and

hormonal problems. It helps ease worry, stress, and irritability and is often drunk in a relaxing tea.

- **St. John's Wort:** Reduces PMS symptoms like cravings, sleeplessness, headaches, bad moods, and tiredness.
- **Turmeric:** This well-known root is good for mending and reducing inflammation. It can help ease the signs of PMS because it contains curcumin.

Herbal medicine is a magical world, and this is just the beginning. You can get help from thousands of plant friends on your path to better reproductive health. There are a lot of herbs and plants that have similar effects, so start by seeing what you can find nearby and following your gut.

Even though herbal medicine is very helpful for people, it shouldn't be used instead of medical advice. If you have any questions, are pregnant, or are taking other drugs, you should talk to your doctor before using any herbs. This is because some herbs can mix with some drugs.

Herbs For Men's Health

For their families, men work hard, both to keep up with the competition and to provide for their families. However, working hard is making worry levels rise. Men deal with worry by picking up bad habits like smoking or drinking too much. These habits can become a permanent part of their lives if they don't have time to exercise or take care of their health. A modern routine like this can lower testosterone levels, which is bad for general health as well as sexual health and fertility.

There are, however, a lot of herbal supplements for men, generally natural herbs for men, that are designed to improve their health and fertility.

Many supplements, both natural and man-made, are sold to men with the claim that they can help them deal with stress and problems like low libido or pregnancy that are becoming more common in men today. So it looks like picking the best pills for men is going to be hard. These are some of the natural herbs and healthy habits I think guys can use to improve their health.

- Live a healthy life. As a nutritionist, I recommend a healthy life that includes:
- It means eating natural, healthy food on a daily basis.
- Keeping up good health habits, like staying away from drugs and booze and smoking
- Getting at least seven to eight hours of sleep every night
- Working out or moving regularly to stay healthy and deal with stress

Herbs that are good for men—Many herbs that are good for men have been used for a long time to improve their health, lower their stress, and stop their birth rate from dropping.

Here is my list of the 10 best herbs for men's health:

- **1. Gokhru:** It helps bring about more babies. Wenyi Zhu's research published in the Chemistry, Central Journal in 2017 says that gokhru helps raise testosterone levels.
- **2. Ashwagandha:** Ashwagandha benefits for guys have been known for a long time to boost energy and vigor. People take

it to boost their energy and directly treat long-term stress because it can drop cortisol levels by 28% and help people sleep better. It treats high blood pressure and diabetes by lowering glucose and blood pressure. These are both causes and effects of stress, which is why it is considered an important herb for guys.

- **3. Safed Musli:** This plant boosts metabolism by sending more blood to the genitalia and making you stronger.

- **4. Sheila Jeet:** This is an old herb for men that helps them act better and get pregnant.

- 5. **Kaunch Beej Extract:** As the name suggests, Kaunch Beej Extract can help men's libido and sexual function.

- 6. **MacaRoot:** This natural root gives you more energy, stamina, and sports performance. It also makes you more fertile and fixes sexual problems like erectile dysfunction (ED) to make you want to be sexual and to boost your immune system.

- **7. Saw palmetto:** This plant can help reduce the signs of an enlarged prostate and manage benign prostate hyperplasia (BPH), both of which are common health problems in older men. It helps you relax, and because it's a diuretic, it keeps you from holding on to pee.

- **8. Yohimbe:** Yohimbe is one of the best herbs for men because it is said to improve blood flow to the erectile muscles, which can help with both physical and mental impotence.

- **9. Ginseng:** Ginseng is one of the best-known herbs for guys that can help increase libido, improve sexual performance, fix erectile dysfunction, and make sperm better.

- **10. Tongkat ali:** As a supplement for men, tongkat ali is one of the few herbs that has one of the strongest hormone-boosting and testosterone-boosting effects of all the plants used. It's also one of the best natural vitamins for men who have trouble getting or keeping an erection.

Because some of these natural herbs are hard to find or can't be eaten every day, I strongly suggest that all men take herbal supplements on a daily basis to help improve their health.

Men don't like to talk about their health and pregnancy problems, so it's important to know how to use the best supplements for men to fix important health problems. These supplements should be made from safe natural herbs for men that don't have any side effects, unlike chemical supplements for men. When it comes to getting healthy and fit, remember that a better lifestyle and the use of the right herbs for men in the form of the best supplements for men can do the trick.

Great herbs for kids, plus tips on how to get them to eat them.

Good things like happiness, wonder, fun, and laughter are drawn to kids, but sometimes bad things like bugs (both real and imaginary) are drawn to them too. Anyone who has sent a kid to preschool, kindergarten, or school knows that they seem to catch everything in the first year. As a new parent, you may not get enough sleep and your immune system may be weaker, so you also catch everything!

When picking herbs for kids, things to think about

Kids and plants are actually very friendly with each other. Herbs seem to work really well for kids, but there are a few things to keep in mind;

- Kids aren't just little people. First, you need to think about safety. They are still growing, so you should keep in mind that their livers are very small and need to be processed and cleaned out. It is also very important to use the right amounts of herbs and pick the right ones.

- It's important to follow through; it's not just a one-dose thing. So often, it's important to think about taste.

- Children seem to have very special health problems (like immune, skin, etc.), so it's also important to keep this in mind.

How to begin

It can be scary to pick out herbs for kids, but keep in mind that high-dose herbs are not the best place to start. Since kids are smaller and still growing, you should use plants with a better safety profile. For example, herbs that help the liver should be given in very small amounts to kids.

When picking herbs for kids, it's also important to know if anyone in your family is allergic to plants. Herbal items can make some people sick. Always start with a small amount to see if you have any reactions. If you do, stop right away if you see anything, like a rash or trouble breathing.

How to get children to take herbs

We made our range with the idea that our own kids would actually want to take it, because we know how annoying it is to buy something and then leave it on the shelf.

If you need more help, here are some simple tricks you can use to get your kids to eat herbs:

- Mix them with Barkers blueberry syrup
- Blend them with other foods
- Put them in juice
- Put them in jelly or gummy bears.
- Turn them into "chocolates"

Figuring out how much to give kids

In plant medicine, Young's Formula can be used to figure out the right dose of medicine for kids, also known as the pediatric dose. If you have an adult formula that would work for a child, this is a great way to figure out what to give your little ones.

For instance, this is how you would figure out the dose for a six-year-old child:

Young's Formula

$$\text{Adult Dose} \times \left(\frac{\text{Age}}{\text{Age} + 12} \right) = \text{Child Dose}$$

Example: You want to work out the dose for a 6 year old child

$$10\,\text{ml} \times \left(\frac{6}{6 + 12} \right) = 3.3\,\text{ml}$$

1. Chamomile flower

One of the best known herbs for kids is chamomile. People often think of kids when they hear this because it's safe and kids love the taste.

It can be used for many things:

- Helping people who have trouble sleeping or staying asleep
- Feeling calm and restless
- Help with mood
- Stressed, worried, angry, or nervous
- Skin inflammation or eczema caused by stress
- An upset or swollen digestive system, gums, or mucous membranes
- Children who have diarrhea: Add chamomile tea to chia seeds or flax seeds to help "bind" an upset stomach.

Studies in people have shown that chamomile:

114

- Using essential oils through inhaling can help calm you down and improve your mood.

- Infusions or tea can help you get a good night's sleep.

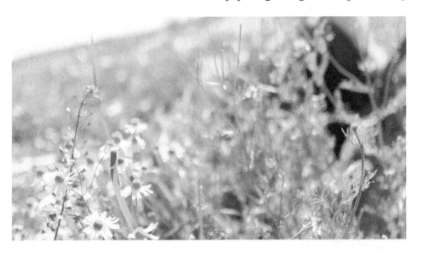

How to use it with kids:

- 1 to 3 cups of chamomile tea every day

- You can take Glycetract up to three times a day to ease your symptoms.

- Putting oil in the steamer at night

- Kids can make a drink with a handful of fresh chamomile.

- Chamomile's azulene components can help soothe sensitive skin and can be mixed with oil to make a balm or cream. This can work a little better than a 0.5% hydrocortisone cream.

Most people think that chamomile is safe for kids, but people who are allergic to plants in the Asteraceae family should stay away from it. Chamomile and fennel seeds are also good for babies who have colic.

We made our Kids Rest and Calm with the right amount of chamomile glycetract and Californian poppy glycetract to help kids from birth. This mixture is very useful because it helps the digestive and nervous systems, and it's especially helpful when little ones are having trouble sleeping.

2. Balm for lemons

Lemon balm is a well-known plant that can help with sleep and mood. It is also sometimes called the "happiness plant" because it can make you feel calm and relaxed. Lemon balm is a safe plant that is great for kids. For now, there are no known side effects.

How to use it with kids:

- Not able to sleep or sleep problems
- Being restless and hyperactive
- Worry, anxiety, jitters, and restlessness
- It helps you concentrate.
- Antiviral: a cream that is put on the skin to treat cold sores
- Analgesic and antispasmodic (reduces pain and spasms) for gut problems like upset stomach, colic, and constipation
- It tastes good when mixed with chamomile and fennel seed.

Researchers have found that seven-year-olds who had a dental exam felt less anxious after using lemon balm. This is good to know because a lot of people, especially kids, have a hard time at the dentist. That's why it's great to have some herbs for kids on hand to make everyday life a little easier.

How to get kids to use lemon balm:

- One teaspoon of lemon balm mixed with 150 milliliters of hot water can be drunk up to three times a day.

- To make a simple syrup, stew fresh or dried lemon balm in water until it cools down. Strain the syrup and add sugar or another sweetener. Kids can take half a teaspoon three times a day, with or without water.

- You can use cream on the skin by adding medicine or lemon balm oil.

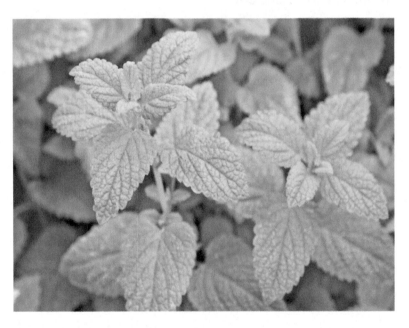

3. Elderberry

Berries are good for you because they taste good and have a lot of vitamins and antioxidants, especially vitamin C. Kids love them. It is safe to eat elderberry, and kids usually don't mind it.

Elderberry is a wonderful plant that is useful all year long. Elderflower can help with seasonal allergies and fevers in the spring and summer. Elderberries grow wild in the cooler months of fall, and you can start using them as a first line of defense to help protect your family.

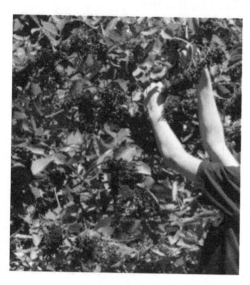

Uses for elderberry

- It's helpful when you first start feeling sick and works great as a first line of defense.
- The effects of elderberries help support the body's natural defenses in general.
- Application of doses often
- Trusted immune system booster for a long time
- Helps fight viruses, inflammation, free radicals, and weak immune systems.
- Rich in antioxidants and anthocyanins, which protect against oxidative stress in a big way

- It has a lot of quercetin and rutin, which can help with pain and swelling.

When used with kids:

- Elderberry mash with warm or cool water
- Elderberry liquor that has been frozen into ice cubes or blocks
- Gummies with elderberries
- Tincture of elderberries
- Tea with elderberries

Elderberry is great for kids who "catch" everything and get sick all the time in the winter. When you start blackberry when the seasons change in the fall, it can help you become stronger. This is why our Immunity Tonic is great for kids, especially when it's cold outside.

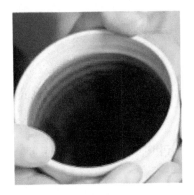

4. Propolis

When you think of "herbs for kids," propolis might not be the first thing that comes to mind, but it is very good at helping the immune system. You can also tell your kids a cool story about how the bees helped make this, which might help them follow through! Our Defense Elixir has propolis in it.

In professional settings, propolis has been used to help with

- Sudden middle ear pain
- Bronchitis with fever
- Sudden respiratory attack
- Sore throat and tonsillitis
- Sudden, stuffy noses
- Acute upper respiratory infections and how to avoid them

Children who seem to get ear and throat problems over and over again can benefit from propolis. Propane should be taken by kids in the following ways:

- Mouthwash
- You can drink Vira Defense Elixir with juice, soda, or lemon and honey.
- Added honey

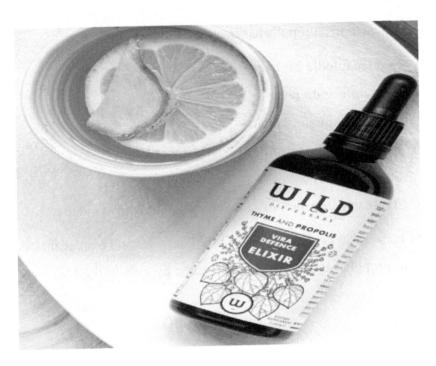

5. Ginger

Kids might not be the best fit for this plant or herb because it can be "hot or spicy," but it can really help with stomachaches and road sickness. The root or rhizome is what is used. It has about 1% to 4% volatile oils, which are what give ginger its strong smell and taste and also hold the active ingredients. Ginger is thought to be a safe plant medicine for kids that doesn't have many side effects.

Here are some ways that kids can use ginger:

- Lemon, honey, or ginger drinks or ice blocks you make yourself
- Ginger candies that you can get at a health food shop and bring with you on long trips
- Ginger jam, pickled ginger, and ginger drink

- A ginger drink
- Up to three cups of fresh ginger tea a day

Kids can get help from Ginger with:

- Feeling sick while moving
- Getting seasick
- Being sick and throwing up
- To make things warmer
- Joint and muscle pain and soreness, as well as stomach pains

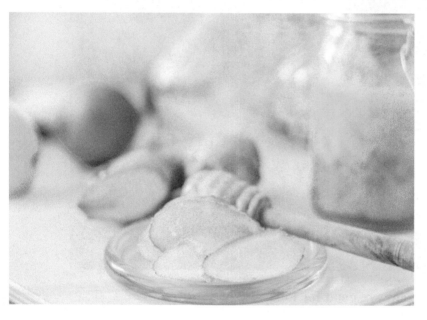

6. Seeds of fennel

For small babies who are nursing and have problems with stomach cramps and gas, fennel seeds may help. The main ingredients in fennel seeds are volatile oil, flavonoids, calcium, and potassium. Lots of kids take them to help with gas and acid, and they also work as a carminative, which means they calm the stomach and bowels.

What it's good for:

- Moms can drink fennel seed tea throughout the day to pass on the health benefits to their babies through breast milk.
- The baby can also be given a cold infusion after being fed. For babies under 5 months, start with 5 drops.
- Using fennel seed in tea or other drinks is a safe way to get its health benefits.

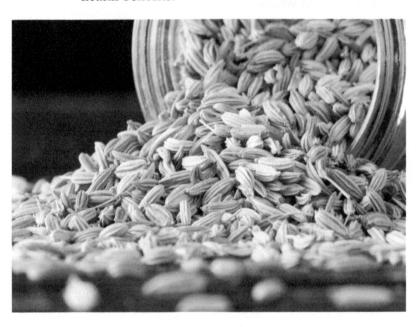

Why greens are good for kids

Kids can improve their health and well-being at home by working with plants. It also helps them understand what is going on in their bodies. If they know that elderberry can help with colds and illnesses, they can ask for it when they think they need it. If they are having trouble sleeping or having anxious thoughts, they can ask for chamomile. In addition to giving them control over their own health problems, it also lets them help themselves.

Chapter 6
Cooking Herbs for Your Kitchen

It's important to have cooking herbs on hand. They do a lot to make your food taste great, along with cooking spices. A little extra flavor makes any food better!

This important list of herbs has all the best kinds you need to know about. When you look at recipes, you'll see these herbs used over and over again.

It's how to use each flower, what it tastes like, where it comes from, and whether it's fresh or dried.

When you cook, herbs are different parts of a plant, usually the leaves or flowers, that are used to make food taste better. Either fresh or dried, they can be used. They are usually sold whole, but sometimes they are chopped or flaked first. Herbs can be used as a decoration or added at different times during cooking.

Spices are like herbs, but they are made from different parts of the plant. In this case, a spice would be anything that isn't a leaf, like seeds, roots, etc.

Herbs: Fresh vs. Dried

You can usually find cooking herbs in both fresh and dried forms. A lot of the time, fresh herbs are better for cooking, but there are times when dried herbs are better. How can you choose the best one for your recipes? Here are some things you should know about each.

- **Fresh Herbs:** These are just herbs that are brand new and come straight from the plant. They are more fragile than dried ones, but overall they are better. They taste the most like nature, but they quickly lose their freshness and strength. Most of the time, fresh herbs should be added near the end of cooking. They work best as decorations or for adding flavor at the last minute.

- **Dried herbs:** These can be kept in the pantry for a long time because they last longer. It's also because their flavors are stronger, you won't have to add as much to your meals. You can also cook with dried herbs for a long time.

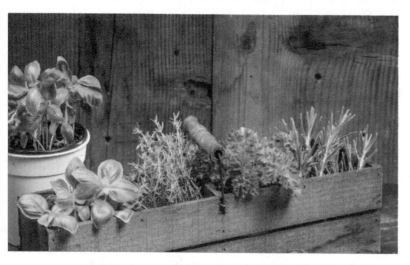

List of Cooking Herbs (A–Z)

This list of popular cooking herbs will teach you everything you need to know to use them like a pro. Buy a lot of dried herbs that you use often and fresh herbs that you use in recipes every week.

Basil

Basil is related to mint, but it tastes more like dirt. There are hints of mint in the taste, along with black pepper and a general herbaceous smell. While some types of basil have a stronger "spiciness" (peppery taste), most people in North America use sweet basil. A lot of people know it as the base for pesto, and it's a key part of any Caprese salad. You can cook it or just put it on top of a lot of Italian recipes.

- When to use it: To give any dish a unique herbaceous and slightly sweet taste. It goes well with soups, meats, Italian and Mediterranean food, and you can use it as a garnish on your favorite spicy dishes.
- Basil recipes: Caprese Stuffed Salmon, Basil Walnut Pesto, and Creamy Basil Chicken

Bay Leaf

The Laurel tree grows bay leaves, which are a leafy vegetable. Often, these are added to soups, stews, and sauces while they are still cooking to give them a slightly sour, almost minty taste that cuts through any richness. Before serving, whole bay leaves should be taken out of the dish, not eaten.

- When to use it: To add a hint of herbiness to meals and keep heavy, rich recipes from being too much.
- Italy Wedding Soup, Instant Pot Ham and Bean Soup, and Homemade Marinara Sauce are all recipes that use bay leaves.

Cilantro

The coriander plant's leaves are used to make cilantro. It is related to parsley. Some people really like this herb, while others really dislike it. It tastes bright and fresh, with hints of citrus and pepper. It's popular in Mexican food and a lot of other types of food too. The best cilantro is fresh cilantro because it tastes and smells the best. It turns dull after being cooked for too long, so add it to recipes near the end of the cooking time or as a garnish.

- It should be used to give food a new taste, usually as a finishing garnish or topping. It tastes great with Mexican, Indian, and Mediterranean food.
- Cilantro and lime recipes, air-fried cilantro lime salmon, and chimichurri sauce

Dill

The celery family has dill, which looks like a feathery green plant. It is also known as dill leaves or dill weed. It makes the food taste fresh, earthy, and a little sweet, almost like licorice but not bitter. Spices like dill pickles, ranch dressing, and potato salad are known to taste good with it. It tastes better when it's fresh and not cooked, or when it's used as a topping. It goes well with vegetables that are cool and refreshing, and it's common in Middle Eastern cooking.

- When to use it: To make cold foods, dips, and other things taste lighter and crisper. It goes well with yogurt, fish, cucumbers, and spreads that are creamy.
- Refrigerator pickles, chicken salad sandwiches, cucumber sandwiches, and more are all recipes that use dill.

Marjoram

Oregano and marjoram are both from the same family, but marjoram is much softer. It tastes fresh and tangy, and it's a bit bitter and sweet at the same time.

- When to use it: To give meat meals, fall recipes, soups, and pastas a citrusy heat.
- Crockpot cabbage roll soup and turkey stuffing are two recipes that use marjoram.

Mint

Most of us quickly think of mint as having a fresh, cool taste in our mouths because of the menthol in it. It tastes slightly sweet and goes well with all sorts of foods, whether they are sweet, savory, or hot. It adds a quick burst of sweetness to foods, levels out spicy foods, and can be used as a garnish to finish off meals.

- When to use it: to give recipes a fresh, sweet taste or to make spicy foods taste less spicy. Plus, it can make all of your cold drinks taste a little better!
- Mint recipes: Pitcher Mojitos and Lamb with Mint Yogurt Sauce

Oregano

The oregano plant's leaves are what make oregano. You can use the leaves fresh or dry. It tastes strong, earthy, almost bitter, and slightly sweet from the mint. It's often put on pizza and comes in a lot of Italian pepper mixes.

Not like some herbs, it can be made right into food without losing its effectiveness.

- When to use it: To give savory foods an earthy taste. Some foods that go well with it are Italian, Mediterranean, and Mexican.
- Recipes with oregano: baked mostaciolli, garlic butter steak, and potatoes in an air fryer

Parsley

Little green herbs like parsley are often used to finish off a dish, but they can also be used to cook. It tastes bright and slightly bitter, which makes other tastes more balanced. It also makes anything taste better with a little extra. If you chop it up, you can add it to meat, rice, or vegetable recipes. Also, you can make soups with it and sauces with it that taste great.

- When to use it: To finish off any savory dish with a bright taste and pop of color.
- Baked Italian Chicken, Cheesy Artichoke Bruschetta, and Garlic Parmesan Fries are all recipes that use parsley.

Rosemary

Rosemary is a very colorful plant that smells great and tastes great too. It's slightly flowery and sweet, but it also has a spicy, peppery side. All kinds of food taste amazing and rich after adding it. It can hold up to long cook times to add a lot of taste to food, and it looks great on top too.

- When to use it: To give many foods a rich, woodsy taste. It tastes great with veggies, breads, citrus flavors, meats (like lamb or chicken), and a lot more.
- Rosemary recipes: Rosemary Garlic Steak, Dutch Oven Rosemary Bread, and Garlic Rosemary Turkey Breast

Sage

Sage tastes like a mix of earthiness, fresh eucalyptus, lemony citrus, and a bit of pepper. This strong flavor works well in recipes and goes well with meat meals, sauces, and other rich foods. It works well with spicy and fragrant foods.

- When to use it: To give chicken, vegetables, soups, and pastas a rich, fragrant flavor.
- Sage recipes include roasted butternut squash with sage, sausage stuffing, and brined chicken breast with crispy sage.

Tarragon

This leafy green herb is best known for being used in French cooking. The taste is like licorice or anise and is sweet, salty, and bitter. It's balanced by a freshness that keeps it from being too much. It works best when it's fresh, since dry forms aren't as strong. Take fresh leaves off the stem and cut them up small enough to use in food. If you cook it for too long, it will taste bitter, so do not add it until the very end of cooking.

- Adding a taste of bittersweet flavor to food is how to use it. It tastes good with veggies, seafood, eggs, and rich sauces.

- Apple Ham Frittata, Herbs de Provence, and Cheesy Sausage Stuffed Mushrooms are all recipes that use tarragon.

Thyme

Thyme has a strong green taste with floral undertones that works well with other tastes. This herb is tough enough to hold up while cooking and adds a beautiful, savory warmth to food. You can also add it to a dish when it's almost done cooking.

- When to use it: To give meat, vegetables, soups, and sauces a light and tasty taste.
- Thyme recipes: Lemon salmon on a sheet pan and sautéed carrots with thyme

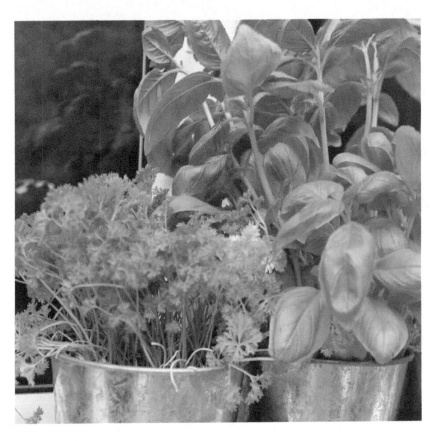

List of Kitchen Herbs

Finally, here are the 12 herbs we talked about for cooking. Make sure you have a lot of these in your kitchen so you're always ready to cook!

- Garlic
- Leaf of Bay
- Coriander
- Dill
- Rosemary
- Mint
- Thyme

- Dill
- Cilantro
- Sage
- Tarragona
- Rosemary

If you want to cook every day, this list of common herbs should be enough. But every once in a while, you might need some more unusual ones. If you're not sure which herbs to use in your recipes or how to find the right one to add the flavor you want, this guide will help you.

Fermenting Herbs

Fermentation is a simple and inexpensive way to make medical herbs more bioavailable and to make fermented foods more therapeutic.

The old art of fermentation has been used to preserve food for thousands of years, but it has become more popular in recent years. Fermentation used to be an old, fusty method often associated with our grandparents from the Great Depression or hippies from the 1960s (think of the so-called Manchurian Mushroom, or kombucha, that was commonly brewed on kitchen benches). Now, many trendy Instagram food and health influencers love it, and there are lots of recipes and ways to do it.

It has a less direct and less well-known link to herbal medicine. Despite this, it is still worth looking into the benefits of this processing method and how it affects herbal products, especially foods and culinary herbs, because more and more evidence points to big benefits in terms of nutrition and phytochemistry.

What does fermentation mean?

While different definitions exist for the same process, fermentation is generally thought of as the metabolic process of breaking down molecules, usually carbohydrates (sugars), into alcohol and/or acids. This is done by the controlled enzymatic actions of bacteria and yeasts. Depending on the product being made and the bacteria that are involved, fermentation can happen either with or without oxygen. During the process, carbon dioxide is often given off. A simpler meaning could be: foods or drinks made by controlling the growth of microbes and changing food parts through the action of enzymes.

Ferments can be "wild," using bacteria and yeasts that are naturally found in the environment, and fermentation usually happens on its own. They can also be "controlled," using certain microbes and temperatures to inoculate the substrate and start the fermentation process, usually with a starter culture. Foods that are usually fermented are dairy (like kefir, cheese, and yogurt), veggies (like kimchi, tempeh, or sauerkraut), and herbal drinks (like kombucha).

History of fermentation

Fermentation has been used for thousands of years to keep food safe. There is proof of fermentation from as early as 8,000 BC. Fermenting foods has been done for a long time in every society and on every continent to keep them safe and make them last longer. This meant that people always had food sources during long, harsh winters and bad growing seasons. This was especially important in ancient times, when food stores were necessary to stay alive. Fermentation protected against hunger and starvation and made sure that an abundance of food was used to its fullest.

Fermented foods and the end of the big microbiome extinction

There are a lot of microbes in the end product because fermentation is mostly caused by the metabolic processes of these bacteria and their growth and reproduction. This is a very important part of how our microbiomes have changed over time; it adds a lot of good bacteria to our food and, by extension, to our guts. But as industrialization has happened and modern food preservation methods that don't need fermentation have come into use, along with a lack of different carbohydrates that our microbiota can access (prebiotics), many of these species have gone extinct in our guts, out of sight and below our awareness3.

Because of appliances like refrigerators, industrial canning, and the mass production of processed and refined foods, some of which contain artificial preservatives, we no longer need fermentation to safely store and preserve foods. As a result, our diet lacks many of the beneficial microbes that our ancestors did, and there is a severe lack of microbial diversity compared to what our ancestors did.

On the other hand, studies have shown that eating more fermented foods can make our gut microbiomes more diverse. This means we have a good way to fix the imbalance and improve our digestive health. Because probiotics support and change the health of the gut and immune system, this may lower inflammation and the chance of a number of long-term illnesses.

Putting herbs through fermentation makes the nutrients more bioavailable.

One of the best and least known benefits of fermentation for people who work with medical herbs is that it makes nutrients and other phytochemicals more bioavailable. This includes the ones in herbs, because the chemicals the plant uses to stop them from breaking down are now broken down, letting the nutrients flow. This is especially interesting for people who work with herbs as food, medicine, or both, because adding culinary herbs to fermented foods can greatly improve both the nutritional value and therapeutic effects of the finished product6, making it even better for you.

In the past few years, there has been a lot of research on how fermentation affects different medicinal herbs. It has been shown that fermentation not only increases certain compounds, especially polyphenols, across a number of species, but it also makes new chemicals in the plants themselves and changes their microbiomes. Similarly, fermenting certain herbs with certain cultures has been shown to make them more bioavailable and improve their healing properties. For example, the Chinese plant Danshen and ginseng can be made more bioavailable.

Scientists looked at how fermenting Basil (Ocimum basilicum) and Peppermint (Mentha x piperita) with the probiotic species Lactobacillus plantarum affected how bioavailable and digestible the plants were. This lab experiment looked at the amounts of phenolic compounds and flavonoids in dried and fermented plants compared to fresh plants. It found big differences in the antioxidant activity and bioavailability between the groups, with the fermented product being better than the fresh herbs.

Looked at the natural microbiomes of two different Asteraceae species (Matricaria chamomilla and Calendula officinalis). It gave us new ideas about how fermentation might change the microbiomes of the herbs themselves. Both the endospheres and exospheres of the plants were looked at before and after fermentation in this study. It was discovered that the leaves of each plant naturally have different groups of microbes that are specific to that herb and to the place where it is grown. These groups changed a lot during the six-week fermentation process. The writers think that this is probably a second benefit of fermented medicinal plants that happens at the same time as their good phytochemical profiles and could make their healing effects even stronger.

What this means for herbal medicine and healthy foods

A lot of herbs that are used in cooking can also be used to treat health problems, which is something we all know. For example, many herbs in the Lamiaceae family that are used in cooking and foods—for example, Thyme (Thymus vulgaris), Rosemary (Rosmarinus officinalis), Sage (Salvia officinalis), Lemonbalm (Melissa officinalis), Lavender (Lavandula officinalis), Mint (Mentha piperita), Oregano (Oreganum officinale), and Basil (Ocimum basilicum)—are also very good at killing food-borne pathogenic microbes and can help to keep food fresh. These herbs are known for their ability to reduce inflammation, and almost all of them will help your digestive system work better and break down food faster.

In the same way, medicinal members of other plant groups have been used for thousands of years in both cooking and medicine. Many plants, like

138

turmeric (Curcuma longa), ginger (Zingiber officinale), chili (Capsicum anuum), parsley (Petroselinum crispum), and coriander (Coriandrum sativum), have been used for a long time in pickled foods all over the world. Again, all of these go well with the tastes of different fermented foods that are easy to include in modern diets and can please modern tastes.

There isn't a lot of research on fermentation and how it can improve bioavailability for many of these herbs, but based on the research that has been done and the fact that they have been used traditionally in fermented foods, it makes sense to assume that the fermentation process will likely improve the bioavailability of not only their macronutrients but also many of their phytochemicals. Ginger, for instance, has many phenolic chemicals that give it many of its health benefits. These include gingerols, paradols, zingerols, and others. Researchers have found that fermenting other herbs increases the amount of phenolics they contain. This could also explain some of the traditional health benefits people say ginger beer has.

Spices like ginger, chili, and other strong flavors are often added to kimchi to make it taste better. There are many classic and modern recipes that use sauerkraut with coriander, ginger, oregano, juniper berries, caraway seeds, parsley, and juniper berries. Fermenting herbal teas can make probiotic health drinks. Ginger beer's long-lasting popularity shows how tasty it is and how easy it is to make10. Similarly, kombucha's rising popularity and widespread availability in fridges in cafes, restaurants, and supermarkets, despite its differing health benefits, shows that people are becoming more aware of fermented foods and drinks in the 21st century.

To sum up, fermentation is a simple, low-cost, and underrated way to improve the health benefits of many of our most famous medicinal herbs, especially those that can also be used in cooking. Even though more research needs to be done before we can say for sure, adding herbs to fermented foods and, by extension, to our diets may help make these herbs more bioavailable and therapeutic, lower levels of anti-nutrients, and almost certainly help with reducing inflammation, increasing the diversity of the microbiome, and supporting digestion, immune health, and overall health.

Chapter 7

How To Plan A Garden – Expert Layout And Planting Advice

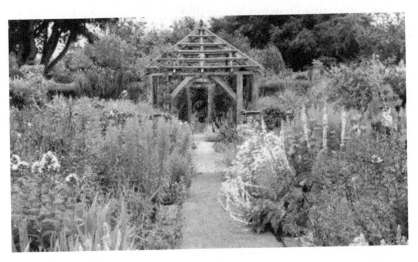

Want to know how to make a garden plan? It's fun to make an outdoor place that fits in with its surroundings and your home the way you want it to.

There are many garden ideas out there, whether you want it to be a place to eat, relax, host, and play, or you just want to add all your favorite flowers and plants.

But there's no doubt that making plans for a yard is also hard. As the years go by and the plants grow, a garden changes, so it's important to plan for both the present and the future.

This information from experts can help you with all parts of planning a plot, from ideas for garden decor to planting guides and more.

How do I start making plans for my garden?

As you start to plan your yard, you should think about what you want to do there and how you want it to look.

A garden's main goal might be to grow flowers, shrubs, and trees, along with maybe some veggies and fruit. It could also be used for something else.

A lot of gardens are used as public places where large groups of family or friends can gather regularly to rest or eat. There are many options for dining outside these days, so there is something for every yard, no matter how big or small it is.

If your outdoor space has an awkward slope, which is notoriously hard to plan around, here are some clever sloping garden ideas that can help. It's also possible that you have a yard with many levels or that you want to make one.

At this early stage, make a list of all the functions you want the garden to have. This will help you figure out how to divide up the room in your layout so that each function can happen easily.

Right now, you should also be thinking about the style of garden you want to have. Should it be standard or new? Are you going to get ideas from formal Japanese gardens or from more casual home gardens? Or do you want to make your yard look more formal?

There are lots of different looks that can fit different styles and that you might also like because of where you live and what that looks like.

How to Make a Garden Plan

Pick out the plants that will do best in your yard first.

It's helpful to look at your yard and where you live to see what plants will do well there before you start planning your garden.

First, take some time to look at your yard during the day. Take a look at the places you want to put your garden and write down if they get sun every three hours, at 9 am, noon, 3 pm, and 6 pm. This will help you decide where in your yard to put plants that will grow in shade, part-shade, or full sun.

Also, you should know what hardiness zone you live in. There are nine hardiness zones in the United States. Each one is based on the temperature of that area. The hardiness zone tells you what kinds of plants do well and don't do well in a certain place. Use a hardiness zone map to find out where you live.

Finding out what kind of soil you have will also help you choose the right plants for your yard or figure out how to feed the soil so the plants can grow well. The best soil for most plants is slightly acidic, with a pH level of about 6-7. However, some plants do better in neutral or slightly alkaline soil.

You can use things you already have to do a simple test at home to find out how basic acidic or alkaline your soil is.

To find out how acidic your dirt is:

- Take a sample of the soil from one or more of your gardens.
- Put in 1/2 cup of water first, then 1/2 cup of baking soda.

It's acidic if the dirt fizzes.

To find out how alkaline your dirt is:

- Take a sample of the soil from one or more of your gardens.
- Put half a cup of water into the sample and then half a cup of white vinegar into it.

There is acid in the earth if it fizzes.

Lastly, you should think about the wildlife in the area (deer love flowers, for example) and decide whether you want to plant a garden that comes back every year, a garden that only blooms once in the summer, or a mix of the two.

Then, think about how it works and how it looks.

There are many trees to choose from, but you can narrow it down based on your needs and preferences.

If you want to keep your privacy, pick plants or trees that grow tall enough to block your view when you choose evergreens for your landscaping. There are tougher plants that won't be easily damaged by balls in your yard if it is next to a playground. There are also plants that can bring in butterflies or keep bugs away.

You might want to divide your garden into zones with areas of lawn, plant-filled beds and borders, and outdoor rooms for eating and relaxing if your garden will also be used as an outdoor living room. This can be the best way to make the most of a space that can be used for more than one thing.

Last, think about how the size and shape of your yard, as well as any hardscaping, will change the way it looks.

How Do You Plan A Garden Layout?

Want to know how to plan the shape of your garden? You could use paper and pencil, which is the old-fashioned way, or you could go digital. In any case, though, having a plan is a good idea at this point.

First, measure the area. Then, make a scaled plan of the garden that you can use to mark where you want the different places to be.

Think about how sunny or shady these spots are and how that affects what you want to do there. Plants or clever trellis ideas can help block the sun, but don't forget about privacy.

You might also want to think about greenhouse plans or other garden buildings.

First, add the hardscape (like walks, paving, and deck ideas) to the plan. Then, mark on both the softscape (like lawns, beds, and borders) you want.

How To Make Plans For Flowerbeds And Pavers

We already told you that beds and borders need to be on your garden plan. But how do you choose how many, how big, where, and what shape they should be?

Borders are used to define the garden's edges, line walks, and go around garden buildings. Beds, which are completely surrounded by grass, dirt, or paving, are where you'll put together plant displays. In some garden types, like traditional gardens, they are the most important part. In modern, low-maintenance gardens, on the other hand, hardscape may take center stage.

You should decide how many and what size plants you want based on the style of garden you want to make and how much time you have to take care of them. Some plants don't need as much care, but in general, more beds and edges mean more work.

It will depend on the style of garden you want to make what shape beds and borders you use.

When it comes to more formal gardening, straight lines are most common. Beds are made up of squares, rectangles, octagons, and even circles. For less formal gardens, think about borders with soft curves. Beds may be round, but soft teardrop shapes are also common.

It's fun to think of flower bed ideas, but keep in mind that what you put in each bed and border should depend on the soil type, the climate in your area, whether the garden is near the coast or exposed to winds, and whether it's in the sun or the shade.

For a more traditional look, they could have just one type of plant, or they could have a mix. If the second option is chosen, plant the fence from back to front and the bed from the middle to the edges.

Trees and evergreens that make a statement all year should come first, then flowering bushes that lose their leaves in the fall, and finally flowers. It's important to think about the shape and size of each plant. If you want to create a natural look, group plants that are different sizes and shapes together.

Pick out a group of materials.

With the right materials and smart garden planting ideas, you can make a garden that fits any style, whether it's modern, cottage, traditional, or formal.

As well as concrete, metal, and wood patio ideas, porcelain and natural limestone patio ideas look great in a modern yard. In more classic gardens, stone, brick, gravel, and wood might all be mixed together.

Think about where the garden is. "Make use of things that are already around you." This will make sure that your garden fits in well with the rest of the scenery.

An easy way to pick the right landscaping materials is to use no more than three different types of hard landscaping materials.

"For a cool, simple look, these should be in neutral colors with small accents of a different color and/or material, like Corten steel or black wood." Choose a warmer color scheme and used bricks for a more classic look.

With smart garden wall ideas, you can connect your yard to the style of your home.

As an example, you could pick bricks that are the same color as a colonial home, granite cobblestones and pea stone to match a normal New England home, slate or wood that matches the roof material, or decking that matches the horizontal wood siding.

"Make sure the design goes well with the property," "If at all possible, the style of the garden should match the house's style and period."

It might be tempting to pave the back of a Victorian house for low-maintenance or plant a cottage garden in a small urban backyard, but the end result might not look right.

Think about how what you want to use will affect the world. "Everyone needs to do their part to stop climate change, and the gardening world could be one of the first to push people to change their habits to be better for the environment,"

The best mix of eco-friendly products for your area will depend on the weather. If you live in a hot, dry place like Southern California or the American Southwest, succulent plants and hardscaping will work better than a lawn and lush flower beds that need a lot of water.

When it comes to places that are milder and rainier, like the Pacific Northwest or the UK, English-style gardens that are mostly kept alive by rain and help add oxygen to the air are better than a lot of man-made hardscaping.

Plan A Garden That Corrects Awkward Proportions

Planning a yard gives you a chance to fix proportion problems. This could be a long, narrow yard or a plot with an odd shape, like a triangle.

To make a small yard look bigger, divide it up into different areas. This will make it look like there is more room. You can also use verticals like green walls, tall, narrow trees, and pergolas to hide borders and give the eye a lot to look at.

When the garden is small, don't think that the plan needs to be as simple as possible. "If you clean up your garden, you can see everything at once, which makes it look smaller,"

"If you put the right size and number of things in the space, like raised garden bed ideas, your eye won't be able to see straight to the back of the garden at once. Instead, it will jump from one thing to the next." This makes the room look bigger than it really is in your mind. Plus, it looks a lot more interesting and appealing.

If you have a long, narrow garden, you don't want people to look straight at the end. To avoid this, divide the space into three squares with different features that draw the eye to different parts of the garden. You could also use a "S" or zigzag pattern to get the same effect.

It's easy to divide a triangle or some other odd shape into different parts that can be round or rectangular. If there's a sharp point in the garden that you don't want to deal with, you could screen it off and use it for a compost pile or storage, or you could put a feature tree there.

"I always try to make the most of the space I have. "Pivot devices" help me connect different spaces." You can change the direction of the axes or the geometry by putting a smaller spot between two bigger areas.

"A sculpture, a big pot, or some other feature can also be used to honor these smaller spaces on their own."

How To Create Interest In A Garden

People really like sensory gardens that have a lot of different colors, shapes, and textures.

There are different types of leaves that I like to divide into groups based on their texture. These groups include "dotty" leaves (Soleirolia soleirolii,

Gypsophila, etc.), spear-like leaves (Astelia, yucca, iris, hemerocallis), and middle, often glossy leaves.

"Keep the list short and use simple mixes of these leaf groups." This really works well in areas that are in the shade.

Use more than just your eyes to help you. When it comes to flowers and flowering bushes, think about how they smell. Sound can be important too. The sound of wind blowing through grass or leaves or the soft trickle of water can make the area more enjoyable.

"I use a lot of light from outside." Pay close attention to how to use lighting in the morning or afternoon. It can change things, especially when it comes through grasses or tall shrubs.

Adding vertical elements, like living wall ideas, and the right hardscaping will make your yard look fuller. It's also important to think about structures like pergolas and focal points like groups of plants and yard sculptures.

Don't make a style where everything is easy to see at once. Ed Oddy says, "Make your garden interesting by screening off some areas to make them seem mysterious and encourage people to explore the whole space."

How to Make a Garden With Shade

In a yard, shade is good. Some gardens are usually shady because of their shape, so they will need plants that do well in that kind of weather. But you should really do your research around areas that face north to make sure they get the right amount of sun and shade.

It can be just as hard to get the hang of a south-facing garden. If your garden doesn't offer any relief, you'll need to find shade so that you can comfortably eat and sit outside.

If you have little kids, you need to think of useful yard shade ideas so they can play without getting too much sun.

Structures and plants, or sometimes a mix of the two, can add shade to the garden and yard around it, making it more fun.

To create a shaded area, you could add pergolas, gazebos, or a roof to a patio or deck. A wall or fence can also provide shade at certain times of the day, which can be useful in a spot you use early in the morning or late at night.

But keep in mind that they won't help when the sun is right above you.

Many structures can be used with plants to add shade, and climbers that flower and smell good make a yard feature look better. But trees and big shrubs can also give a yard the shade it needs.

Other things that can be used to provide shade around the yard are patio umbrellas, awnings, canopies, shade sails, and cabanas.

How to Make a Garden Private

Because of where our homes are, many of us have gardens that our neighbors don't see, especially in cities. However, there are many garden privacy ideas that can help you make your outdoor place feel safe when you're planning it.

Some people might not like it when people outside their yard can see into their garden, so a bush can help block that view. You could also use pleached trees, whose branches are trained to grow on a trellis or some other structure to make a wide sweep of leaves that blocks views into the yard.

You can also use them all over the place instead of planting along the edges.

You can also plant things like bamboo or tall grasses to keep your yard private. Climbers or ivy on a vine or pergola are also pretty and useful ways to block out views.

How To Make A Garden For Vegetables

A vegetable garden, also called a home garden, is important for many people. This kind of plant needs some planning and thought, just like other kinds.

For starters, you should put it somewhere sunny if you can. Instead, choose a spot with more shade if you can't do that. Lettuce, cabbage, and kale are good choices for locations like these.

If you want to grow foods that need to be picked often, it will be easier to keep your vegetable garden close to the house. For watering, put it where the hose can reach or far enough away that you don't mind carrying a watering can.

Putting the compost pile close to the vegetable yard can be a good idea because compost is heavy and you don't want to have to move it over long distances. Keep in mind that putting the compost somewhere with some shade will mean you spend less time adding water to the pile.

When choosing a spot for a vegetable garden, you should think about how much room you have and how many hours you have to care for the plants.

There are also crops that can be grown in pots or very small raised beds because they are more compact than others. On the other hand, deep beds can help you grow more plants in a smaller area.

What kinds of plants should I put together?

One way to keep your garden healthy is to use companion planting, which means putting plants together that do well with each other. Depending on the pair, companion plants can help each other by providing shade, keeping pests away, or making the dirt better.

Here are some common partner plants:

- Cabbage and onions
- Cabbage, beans, peas, and peppers
- Tomato and basil
- Lettuce and cucumbers, dill and mint
- Garlic and most veggies, because it keeps aphids away.

Learn how to make a garden from scratch.

It can be hard to start planning a garden from scratch, whether it's a small garden in the city or a big garden in the country. I believe that good design is all about managing the many different aspects of a garden, such as its size, shape, color, structure, light, dark, charm, strength, sense of place, romance, history, and so on. But once you start, there aren't really any hard and fast rules. Over time, every gardener develops their own set of skills that help them.

The great thing about gardens is that you can watch them grow over many years. Because of this, I believe it is best to keep the plan simple and classic. Then, as you get better at working with the land, you can re-energize the planting and try new things with it over time. When you first start, here are some things to think about.

How to plan a garden

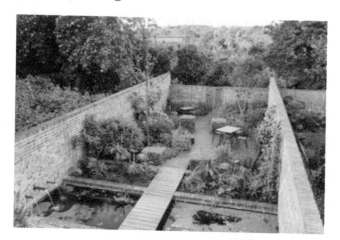

1/17

Make a dream list before you start.

Think about what you need and how you will use your plant before you start. The first thing you should think about is a place to sit with some pretty outdoor chairs. This should be close to the house and, if possible, face southwest.

You might need room for things you use every day, like a clothes line or a place to store toys. Would you like a food garden? How about some room for your kids? You will need compost for any type of yard, and serious gardeners may want a shed.

You should plan where you want to sit in your city garden when you get home from work and whether you want a garden full of plants or one that is easier, with things like water and beautiful paving, and bordered by a wall, a beautiful fence, or plants.

Find out what your garden needs most and stick to a simple plan with one or two "wow" moments if it's small. Plant simple things like grasses or roses with evergreen trees and fill plant pots to the brim with all your favorite seasonal plants.

Take a little more time to picture your garden if it's big. Figure out what goes where and how you can divide the room. Be brave and think about how you can play with size.

Find out where the sun goes down and put your plants so that they get the light of the setting sun.

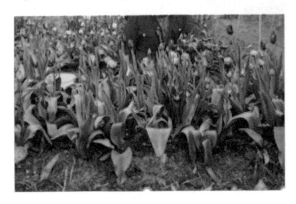

2/17

Think about the soil.

Making sure the soil is ready is the most important thing you can do for your yard. Picture the great soil in Monty Don's yard, and try to get it: not packed down, good drainage, and soft, nutrient-rich soil. It will make your plants happy and healthy for years to come. Two of the first things you need to do to have a great yard are compost and good soil.

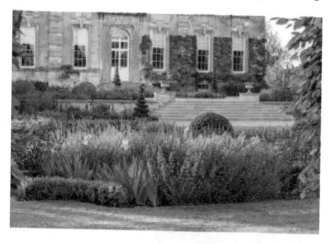

3/17

The formal yard is a style

In a formal garden, symmetry and balance are two of the most important things. Geometric shapes in a simple planting scheme are also very important.

Pick a shape and use it over and over again in the yard, whether it's for flower beds, paths, water, or the space between these things.

Putting shrubbery and plants in pots in the right places will give your garden a nice, clean look that should be easy to keep up.

Don't use too many colors when you plant. For example, use a pale palette of yellow, cream, white, and lime green, or a range of blues, grays, and deep reds. All of these will calm the eye, and nothing else will do.

Cut your trees into formal shapes, like lime, hawthorn, or hornbeam. If your yard is big enough, plant some of these trees farther apart and let them grow on their own.

As we saw above, a formal pool should be very easy. The shape of this pool will be used all over the garden.

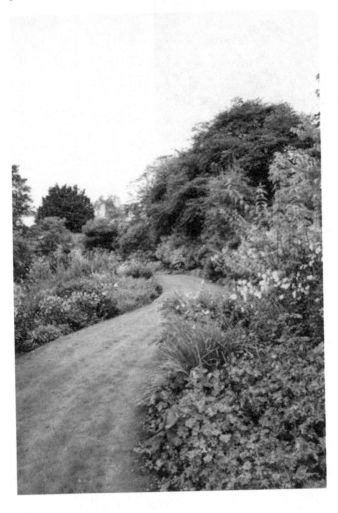

4/17

The garden without rules

In contrast, informal gardens don't have to have straight lines and the same shapes over and over again. They can be wild and free. Eco-friendly materials are used whenever possible, and grassy areas are kept longer and filled with flowers.

There are paths that go through the yard that are shaped like natural borders and are full of grasses, shrubs, roses, perennials, and other plants.

If you have paths, try making shapes that curve and wind around.

Make your yard look like the country by putting poppies and plants like Anthriscus sylvestris 'Ravenswing' and Cenolophium denudatum, which look like the wild umbellifers you can find in the hedgerows.

For a romantic look, let plants grow from seeds along gravel walks and roses climb trees.

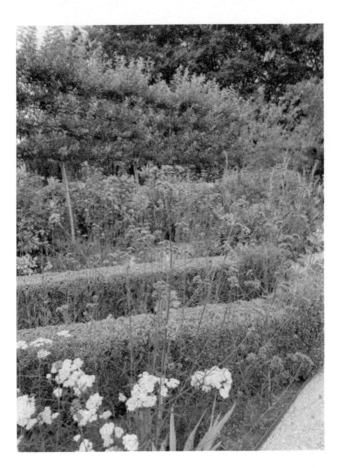

HOW IT WORKS

When you choose a spot to relax in your yard, you need to think about how it will be built. What kind of garden features do you want? A hedge, a fence, bridges, gates, sculptures, planters, or topiary? Think about how less is more if your garden is small. To keep things from getting too crowded, try using only three or five of the great ideas above.

5.Walls, fences, and hedges

If you need a tall hedge for your yard, you should decide if it will be evergreen. If it will be, yew is a great choice. You should be very careful when planting yew because it needs to be able to drain well. If you are planting in heavy soil, you should add at least 200 mm of grit to the hole you made. It also likes to be fed in the winter, so feed it all year long, and in 3–4 years you'll have a good fence. If you want a fence that loses its leaves in the fall, hornbeam does well in clay soil and beech does well in lighter soil. You can also make pretty fences out of Rugosa and other roses.

If your yard has a slope that goes down, it's a good idea to make the most of it by drawing a line where the level changes. After that, you can make another "room" that might have a view of the farmland. The line can be a wall or a bush, and it will probably also block the wind.

So long as your yard slopes up away from the house, it might be best to keep the view open by using short walls and hedging to divide the space.

Putting up hedges or walls that block your view of most of the garden can make a small garden feel bigger. Putting up a mirror at the end of the garden can make it look longer.

Some parts of a structure can be used for decoration only. When you grow roses up arches, they make a yard look more romantic. To make an apple bower, you can also build an arch with a trained crab apple tree on each side. There should be at least 2m of space between each arch's height and width. The flowers of Rosa "Souvenir de la Malmaison" hang down, making it a good rose for an arch.

When you need to stop, gates are great, and the more beautiful they are, the better. If your yard is in the shade, paint your gate a light cream color.

I like "Downpipe" from Farrow & Ball for yard gates, but "String" from them is also nice.

There are lots of different styles and sizes of fences, and they don't always have to block views. A decorative fence might let you still see the scenery beyond.

In the picture, diagonally planted hedges in an Oxfordshire garden make the room feel wider than it really is.

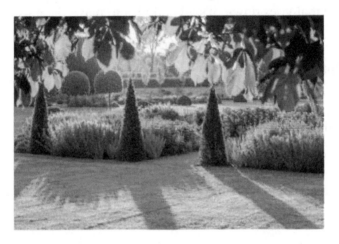

Topiary plants

Topiary is a striking structural feature that is usually found in more formal gardens. It is a good way to make things look balanced. If you run three topiary cones or other shapes down each side of a small yard, it will look great with little work. If your garden is big enough, you can plant them in the yard. If your garden is small, you can plant them in the border, like shown above. The geometry and symmetry will make your yard feel like a safe, comfortable place right away. Most of the time, box and yew are the best plants for topiary. However, Euonymus japonicus, Osmanthus burkwoodii, and Phillyrea angustifolia are also great options.

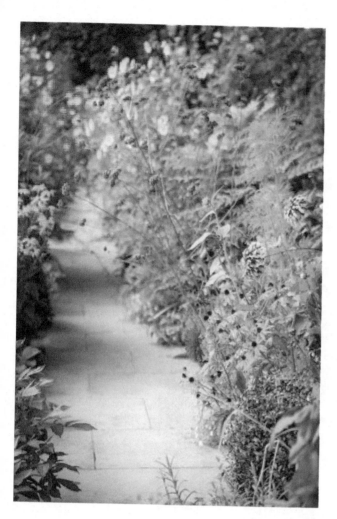

The Ways

It's likely that the hardest parts of landscaping your yard will be the hard parts. Take a look at your house and choose the color of stone or soil that goes best with it. Then, don't use more than three different types of materials. You could pick gravel, stone, and brick, or you could pick gravel, metal, and wood. In most gardens, I like paths made of grass and gravel. But in veggie gardens, I think paths made of brick or very flat breedon gravel are best. Stone is often used around the house, but be

162

careful, it can be slippery! When you're putting out the paths, think about the style of your garden. For a romantic garden, you want soft, wavy shapes. For a more formal garden, you want straight lines and symmetry.

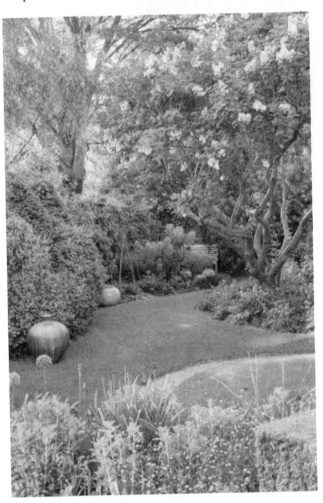

Points of focus

Make the garden even better by adding to its good points. For instance, if you have a beautiful cherry tree or magnolia in your yard, plant spring bulbs around the base of it to draw attention to it. Camassias look beautiful with cherry blossoms that bloom later, and narcissi look great with magnolias. I also love putting flowers and alliums in long grass.

Find something interesting in the distance if you can, and open up the yard to see it. Just be careful not to make a wind tunnel at the same time. Adding an avenue of trees or big bushes around a view will make it look better.

Find ways to make views in the yard itself. As the center of attention, you can make your own urns, wall fountains, seats, troughs, or a single rose, shrub, or tree. Putting these on at night is always a good idea.

Even when they are covered in snow or frost, bridges and pergolas are still important parts of the winter garden because they make it stand out.

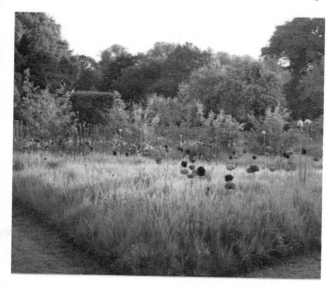

ESSENTIAL PARTS OF THE GARDEN

Plants: grass

It's almost necessary to have a lawn in an English garden, and there's nothing better than a newly mowed lawn to set off all the borders and longer grass areas.

Instead of mowing the grass, why not make a garden that looks like a meadow? You could put bulbs, snowdrops, crocuses, camassias, tulips, alliums, and even roses there. After the first year of planting, the bulbs need to be grown by 50% more each year after that. This is a great way to make a garden that doesn't need much care and also attracts lots of different animals and wildflowers. If you mow in straight lines between the shapes you've made, the area will look neat and natural.

When you want blooms, you need to plant yellow rattle seeds every five to ten years. Yellow rattle is a plant that lives on the roots of grass. In this way, it thins the grass so that there are more plants. For starters, the long grass needs to be scarified in the fall to make bare spots, then the yellow rattle needs to be planted. It needs eight weeks of cold to sprout, and you can plant it again in February. If you can, ask kind friends for seed. In places where the yellow rattle seed hasn't grown yet, you need to plant the seed every year for five years.

Pictured: Angel's home's parterre field, which is filled with tulips and alliums and supported by pillars of cut hornbeam.

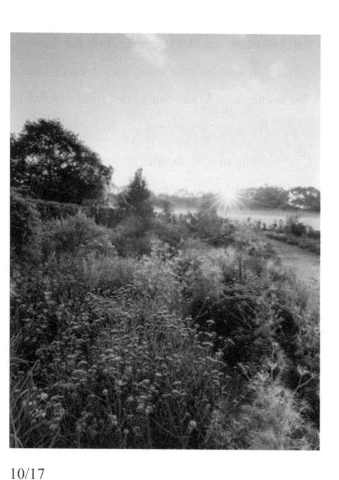

The edges

Start with the front, middle, and back rows as a guide for most borders. The back row needs to be the largest, and the front row needs to be the shortest. Next, pick three perennials that flower at different times of the year for each row. Repeat this process, this time putting the plants in groups of three or five, making sure they are not lined up but instead spread out. It's possible for this to look too neat, so try to give your planting some movement. It doesn't matter if your group runs into a different row.

In between the rows, switch between spikey flowers and round flowers. For romance, add roses, and for interest all year, add a bush like a viburnum that blooms in the winter or a Magnolia stellata that blooms in the spring.

You need a strong base of perennials in your border so that it looks good all year. Then, you can run the stars of each month through them. A tulip in April and an allium in May. To hide the ugly allium leaves, put a perennial with nice leaves, like an astrantia. In June, roses will bloom, and by the middle of July, dahlias will be here.

For the front row, you should use Nepeta, salvias, amsonia, alchemilla mollis, and stachys as reliable filler plants. For the front and middle rows, you should use salvias, astrantias, knautia, or perovskias, and for the gaps between the asters and veronicastrums, you should use campanulas, delphiniums, fennel, and thalictrums.

Don't forget to use shapes and textures that are different from each other in the flower heads and leaves. The Thalictrum 'Elin' plant grows very tall, and so do the Delphinium 'Faust' and 'Elatum'. I also think you should check out the great new Veronicastrum called "Red Arrows."

When you buy plants, try to find ones that have "AGM" (Award of Garden Merit) in their name. It has been tried and tested, so you can be sure it will do well in your yard.

In this picture, you can see a border in Alasdair Cameron's Devon garden. It is made up of grasses, perennials, and taller trees and yew domes.

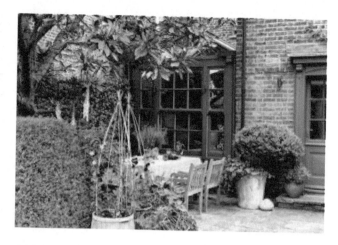

Containers

In a yard, containers are the cherry on top. They are made of rock, wood, clay, metal, terracotta, and stones. They also come in different sizes and shapes. Since plant pots are often put close to the house, pick materials that go with the style of your home. Put the smaller packages together in groups of three.

For smell, I always try to have an evergreen plant like Daphne "Eternal Fragrance" in a pot by the door. Around the outside of this, you can either put spring bulbs or hellebores and euphorbias to make it last. Rosemary 'Miss Jessop's Upright' or 'Tuscan Blue' grown with Erigeron karvinskianus is another easy long-term plant.

You can also put spring bulbs in pots. For example, tulips do better in pots than in borders because they are easier to move and grow again the next year. Wallflowers and tulips look great together. The strong and long-lasting pink tulip "Menton," the white tulip "Jan Reuss," or the "White Triumphator" would look great with the wallflower "Ruby Gem." I put a lot of Narcissus 'Thalia' and Leucojum 'Gravetye Giant' in pots this year, and they flowered all summer. Daffodils and snowdrops are signs of spring.

After the spring bulbs are gone, it's time to think about summer planting. I like to center my arrangements around one plant; Salvia 'Amistad' is the best choice because it grows so well. When I'm in this area, I like to choose verbena, felicias, geraniums, cosmos, orlaya, and diskus. Leave the plant in the middle of the pot but cut off the bottom. This way, the plant's roots will go down instead of out. This means the other plants will have room to grow well. You should feed and remove dead flowers from your summer pots once a week.

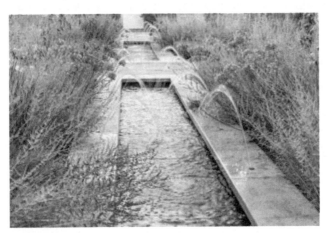

12/17

Water

Not only should every garden have water for the birds, but it also makes the garden feel calmer, and if you live near a road or train track, a pond can help block out the noise.

Water should be simple and the right size for its surroundings. An oval-shaped, very shallow pool with a black-painted brick edge looks great in country settings and is easy to keep clean. It only has to be 200 mm deep. For a more formal yard, long, rectangular pools are always a good choice. With a water grill just below the surface to catch anyone who falls in, raised pools are a good place to sit and keep kids safe.

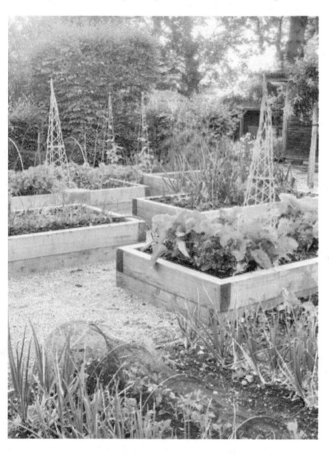

13/17

Fruit, veggie, and herb growing

Plants like sweet peas, runner beans, growing zucchini, gourds, and rows of onions can look just as pretty as roses and bushes. We're all crazy about growing veggies this year, so if you have room in your garden, all your hard work will pay off.

But don't forget how hard the work is. If you don't have much time, like I do, stick with chard, onions, parsley, radishes, lettuce, and rocket. They're pretty much always good.

Most people grow their veggies in raised beds, which you can buy or make yourself (learn how to build a raised bed). The beds should be set up in symmetrical groups of four or six.

You can easily grow a lot of vegetables and herbs in pots or other places if you don't have a vegetable yard. For example, rosemary and sage do well in borders, and thyme grows well through paving.

To grow the best vegetables, keep these simple rules in mind:

- Make sure the soil you use for your veggies is the best it can be.
- For vegetable beds, pick a sunny spot in your yard.
- For raised beds, 1.2 meters is the best width. After that, they can be as long as there is room for.
- To keep the wood safe, it's a good idea to line raised beds with landscaping cloth.
- If you can afford it, irrigation saves a lot of time because you have to water the plants every day.

Pictured are raised beds that give The Light Bar and Dining restaurant a lot of veggies.

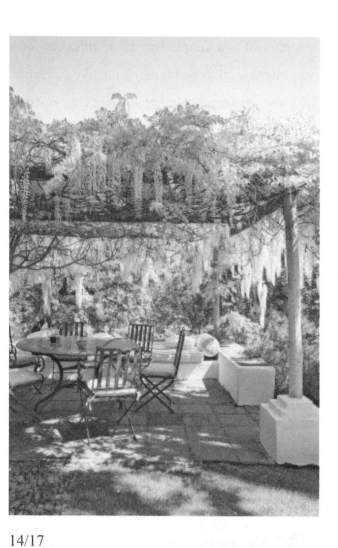

Making a place to sit

The place where you sit and eat should be close to the kitchen and as comfortable as possible. Will there be plants around you or will it be open? Topiary plants like standard wisteria or Phillyrea angustifolia can be used to make a nice natural fence around the area.

Also, think about shade. A parasol is a simple way to do this, but for a more stable, shady spot, you might want to build something like a pergola. Then you might want to grow wisteria to cover it. Wisteria sinensis "Prolific" is good for a pergola because it's easy to trim and bees love it. Wisteria floribunda 'Alba' is a beautiful white one.

Make sure that your table fits well and that there is enough room to move around. Put pots of flowers and geraniums close to where you'll be sitting so that the area smells nice.

Pictured is a pergola wrapped in wisteria.

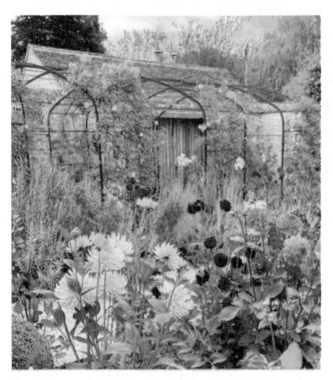

15/17

THE GARDEN OF SENSORY

15. Color

You could add color to the yard in a number of different ways. You might only want one or two colors, like the famous white garden at Sissinghurst. You could also like soft colors, rich jewel tones, or a variety of colors.

Another important thing to think about is what color your house is, especially if you have plants next to or growing up it. It goes with everything, which is one reason why everyone loves soft Cotswold stone. Euphorbias' lime green, golden fennel, Rosa mutabilis, Gleditsia triacanthos 'Sunburst', and any creams and blues look great with Hornton sandstone's orange undertones. Brick can be harder to work with. Red and silver plants look good on brick, like Rosa "Chevy Chase" that spreads out and growing teucrium fruticans. You can also use dark wine colors, and creams and lime greens look great together.

As a general rule, if your border is far away, use strong oranges, reds, and blues to make it look closer. When it comes to edges close to the house, I like to use softer colors. Make sure there is a splash of bright lime green in every border. It looks great.

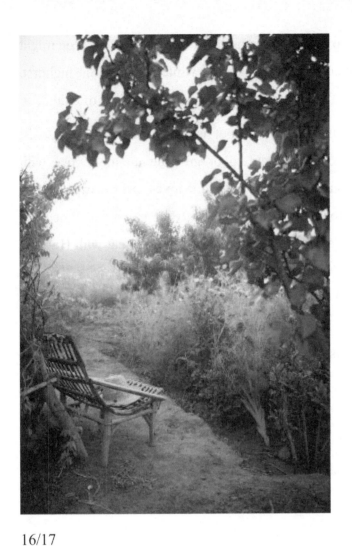

The scent

When I was going down a shady path to a friend's front door after it had rained, I will never forget the wonderful scent of lemon-scented lily of the valley that was wafting up. I wanted to bottle it. Smell is an important part of any yard, so make sure you plan for it.

In any yard, you must have roses, wisteria, honeysuckle, Philadelphus "Belle Etoile" and "Mexican Jewel," Lillium regale, hesperus, and calycanthus. They all smell great. "Mme Alfred Carriere" is one of my favorite roses, but if you asked me to pick a plant based on smell, I'd pick Rosa primula, also known as the incense rose. Along the yard path, it gives off a wonderful incense-like scent. But it's the leaves that smell, not the flower. Calycanthus 'Aphrodite' is one of the most beautiful and fragrant plants, in my opinion.

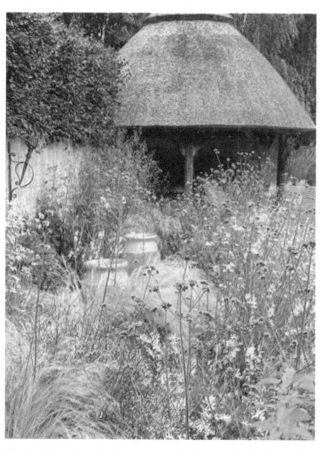

17/17

Texture

One of the most important parts of any yard is texture, but it's easy to forget about. Place your hands over your eyes and look out at your garden. You need stronger forms if it all blends together into a soft mass. If it all seems too heavy, you should put lighter things in other places. Mix a soft grass like Stipa tenuissima with Rosa 'Desdemona', then add more texture with clipped hornbeams inside the softer plants around them, and finally contrast the straight lines of blue salvias with the round, lighter shapes of garnet-colored Knautia macedonica. And there is nothing like seeing different kinds of green plants to really understand how texture works in a yard. The strappy leaves of the Hakonechloa macra plant can be used with Euphorbia "Phrampton Phatty," cornus, and magnolia to make a border with bigger plants.

How to Take Care of Herbs and Grow Herbs From Seed

Herbs for cooking

When it comes to gardening, culinary herbs are probably the most useful because they can be used in so many ways in cooking and baking. Because they have strong flavors, these herbs are usually only used in small amounts to make food taste better and look more interesting.

Types of herbs

There are three types of herbs: annuals, biennials, and perennials.

- **Annuals:** Some plants, like anise, basil, chervil, coriander, and dill, only bloom for one season and then die.

- **Biennials:** Caraway and parsley are biennials, which means they only bloom in the second season.
- **Perennials:** Some perennials, like chives, fennel, lovage, marjoram, mint, tarragon, thyme, and sometimes rosemary (depending on how bad the winter was), survive and grow every year after they get established.

Outside activities

Your herb garden can be separate from your vegetable garden, in a separate area of your yard, or in pots. Additionally, you can put them in flower beds because many herbs are pretty and are great for pollinator gardens.

Size of herb garden

How big your herb garden is will depend on how many and what kinds of herbs you want to grow. An herb garden can be anything from a formal garden with a low-growing hedge around the edges to a few pots outside the kitchen door to make herbs easy to pick.

Place and factors for growing

- Herbs need at least six hours of full sun. In light shade, you can grow chervil, mint, onions, and cilantro.
- Herbs need dirt that doesn't stay soggy. It's likely that drainage is the most important thing for raising herbs. Soils that are too wet won't let herbs grow.
- "Mediterranean" herbs, like lavender, oregano, basil, and thyme, do best where it is warm and dry with light soil.

- Do not add sand to clay soil or to make it drain better. If the soil doesn't drain well, build a raised bed.

- The soil in the bed doesn't need to be very rich in nutrients. When the earth is very fertile, plants tend to make too much leafy greens that don't taste good. Too much fertilizer can lower the amount of vital oil in herb plants and make root and stem rot diseases more likely. Some plants, like chervil, fennel, and lovage, may need a small amount of fertilizer.

- Adding a small amount of compost to clay soil will help it drain better and keep its shape.

- Established flowers can handle dry conditions, but during droughts, they should be given extra water. To keep the earth moist, but not at the base of the plants, mulch can be used.

Sowing seeds for herbs

- You can grow almost any plant from a seed. Sure, there are some cases, like lavender seeds, which can be hard to grow.

- Anise, borage, coriander (cilantro), dill, and fennel do not do well when moved, so plant them straight in the garden.

- To plant seeds, work the soil's surface until it is fine and slightly wet.

- Dig a shallow hole, put the seeds, and then pack the soil down over them. Usually, the finer the seed, the deeper it should be planted, but check the advice on the packet to be sure.

- When you plant fine seeds like oregano or thyme, mix them with sand first to make them spread out more evenly.

- Spray a fine mist of water on plants after you put them.

- You can start basil, parsley, sage, marjoram, and many other herbs indoors and put them outside when it's no longer cold.

Cutting and splitting

- Cuttings and division are two ways to make new herbs plants. When seeds take a long time to sprout, division is the best way to make new plants.

- You can split tarragon, chives, and mint, but lavender needs to be grown from cuttings.

- If you want to make a cutting, start the plant growing in the spring or early summer. Cut a three- to four-inch long stem that is healthy and not yet hard. The bottom end should have its leaves and stems cut off. It should then be dipped in rooting hormone and put in a moist growing medium like vermiculite or peat and perlite mix. Use plastic wrap to cover the pot so that it doesn't touch the plant. Every day while the cutting grows roots, mist the soil. When the new leaves start to grow, you'll know it has roots.

Getting flower seeds ready to plant next year

As the seed heads turn from green to brown or gray, they are ready to be picked. That's because seeds dry out more slowly than leaves. For bigger seeds, it can take up to two weeks. Put the seed heads on paper or cloth. When the seeds are almost dry, gently rub them between your hands to get rid of the dirt and hulls. Clean seed should be spread out on cloth or paper in thin layers until it is quite dry.

If you hang the whole plant upside down in a paper bag, the seeds will dry out too. The bag will catch the seeds as they dry out and fall off the pod.

Herbs for the winter

Winter care should be given to perennial and biennial flowers. A lot of herbs have weak roots, which means they can be heaved out of the ground when the ground freezes and thaws. To protect the plants, lay down 4 inches of straw, oak leaves, or evergreen boughs as mulch. In early winter, after the ground has frozen, put down the mulch. Don't take away the mulch until early spring, when the plants start to grow. If you take them down too soon, the frost could hurt them.

It is possible to bring evergreen herbs like rosemary inside for the winter, but it can be tricky. They do not like it when it is hot and dry inside, which is what most houses are like when the heat is on. The herbs should be left outside in a protected area until the temperatures drop into the low forties at night. After that, bring them inside and put them somewhere cool and out of the way of air. Put them somewhere that will get strong straight sunlight or under "cool white" fluorescent lights. Lessen how often you water; only water when the potting mix feels dry. Check for bugs like spider mites and aphids every so often and treat them if you find any. Next spring, when there is no longer a chance of a hard frost, bring them back outside.

Chapter 8
Foraging for Food and Medicine: Wild Edibles

Fireflies that flash green light and trees that hang low with lush leaves make the wild world magical. Sometimes I wish I had set up a timelapse camera to record the slow but steady march of the plants as they stretch and creep, taking over our yards and gardens in their seasonal victory. What started in early spring with the first green sprigs is now the plant kingdom's full-on attempt to take over the world, and I love it more than anything.

It shows that our well-kept and "civilized" landscape is only temporary, and that the plants are ready to take back their rightful place on the world at any time. However, it also serves as a reminder that we are a part of nature. Everything we need is all around us, growing in cracks in the sidewalk, climbing over trees, and trying to take over our yard plots.

A long time ago, before our food system became organized, our ancestors got their food by searching for it in the wild. Explorers who came to our country were able to stay alive because the locals taught them how to grow crops and identify plants that were edible or medicinal. Many of our grandparents and great-grandparents lived off of food they found along the roads, in meadows, woods, and fields in their own areas, even during the Great Depression.

With how easy and convenient food stores are now, many of us have forgotten this. Backyard gardens have also become less popular over the last few decades. But as the cost of food goes up and people become more interested in alternate health, independence is coming back. More people are farming these days. And there is an increased interest in finding, gathering, harvesting, and cooking foods that grow in our environment.

Why would we want to go hunting now that there is so much food around? Many things lead to this. Some people have found that medicines found in nature work better, are safer, or cause fewer side effects than drugs. A lot of us want to bring back the knowledge of our ancestors. Some people like eating wild foods because they are healthy, don't contain pesticides, and haven't been genetically changed. For some, the trip itself is very satisfying. A walk through a forest, up a hill, or even in your own backyard can lead you to seeds, stems, flowers, leaves, fruits, and roots that you can eat.

No matter what your reason is for paying attention to the plants around you, you will quickly learn that the "weeds" you walk by every day may be there for a reason other than getting in the way. In your study, you may find that health and plenty are already in the natural world. We just need to know how to get to them. They come to us in the form of a wealth of wild plants that we can eat!

At Azure, we believe that using wild plants for food and medicine is an important part of living a healthy, happy life. It's fun to learn how to recognize and use the plants that grow in your yard. We are amazed at how wise and kind our Creator is, and the more we learn, the more we learn.

Here are some wild plants that you can eat or use as medicine that you can find in most of our country. We chose to talk about a few plants that are commonly thought of as "weeds" because they grow wherever you look. We didn't include local species that are rare or have been overfished.

Note: Please be careful when gathering because many plants that look like edible ones are actually poisonous. Plant recognition books can teach you a lot, but if you're still not sure, talk to an experienced herbalist or botanist before eating any wild plants. However, if you learn how to correctly identify plants, you will have more things to choose from and a backup plan in case something goes wrong.

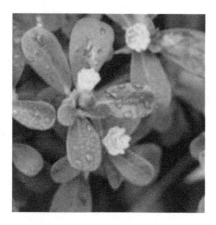

Purslane: As the name suggests, purslane is a leafy green succulent plant that can grow anywhere, even in harsh circumstances. It does well in cracks in the ground, empty lots, along the sides of roads, in yards, and in old garden plots. One of the most nutrient-dense plants in the world is purslane. It has the most omega-3 fatty acids of any plant and vitamins A, C, and E, which are good for your eyes, immune system, and cells. There is a lot of calcium, magnesium, zinc, and iron in it. This delicious leafy green tastes sour and salty and goes well in salads, sandwiches, sautés, and even smoothies. This plant's leaves can be eaten raw, cooked, or spicy. If you want to treat colds and coughs with tea, you can use purslane. If you have a cut or burn, you can use pumice.

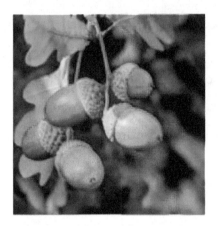

Acorns: Most of us are familiar with acorns, which are the seeds of an oak tree. They are high in calories, which makes them a great food to eat. You should mash and then rinse the acorn meat to get rid of the bitter chemicals that are in them before you use it for flour or meal. They can also find other nuts, which is pretty cool. You can gather nuts from hickory, walnut, chestnut, beech, and even pine trees. These nuts are high in carbs, protein, and fat, which gives you energy and calories.

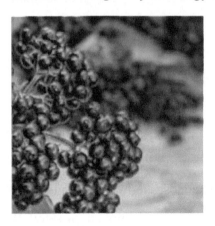

Elderberries, or Sambucus spp: are blue to purple-black berries that grow wild in many parts of the US. One of the best natural ways to get vitamin A, thiamine, calcium, and niacin is from these foods. There are many kinds of elderberries, and the ones that are safe to eat rely on how much hydrocyanic acid (a bitter toxin) they have. The more bitter the taste, the more poison they have. The leaves and bark have more poison than the other parts of the plant, so you shouldn't eat them. Cook or make a syrup with the ripe berries before you eat them. Elderberries are great for making jams, jellies, wines, and pie fillings. Elderberry juice is often used as a cough syrup, to boost the immune system, and to treat cold symptoms. Poultices and ointments made from elderberries are good for treating skin problems.

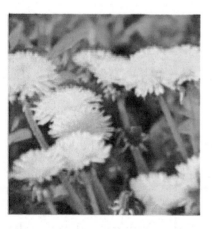

Dandelion (Taraxacum officinale): Wild dandelions are often thought of as an unwanted weed that grows in yards or along roadsides, but they are good for the soil and can be eaten or used as medicine. Any part of a dandelion can be used. From the flowers, you can make a salve. From the leaves, which are high in vitamins A and K, you can make pesto. And from the roots, you can make dandelion coffee. Young leaves taste better and are less bitter. You can eat them raw or add them to recipes. For better taste, boil the leaves and roots that are fully grown before eating them. As a snack, you can eat the bright yellow flower heads raw. You can also add them to a salad for color or fry them as a side dish. People believe that dandelion can help cleanse and detoxify the body, lower inflammation, and protect against a number of chronic illnesses. Vitamins A, C, K, and folate are all found in good amounts. It has a lot of calcium, magnesium, and iron.

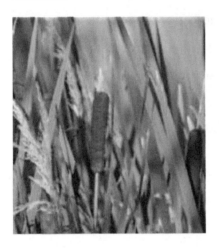

Cattails (Typha spp.): are tall plants that look like reeds. They are one of the most useful wild plants for food and can be found in big groups along the edges of marsh and freshwater areas all over the US. You can eat the whole plant, and it's a great way to get calories. You can eat the tender leaves raw or sautéed in the spring. Late spring's yellow pollen can be used instead of or along with flour. Its flower spike looks a lot like corn on the cob, which you might also like to eat. You could dry the fluffy seeds that make up the spike if you need something to start a fire.

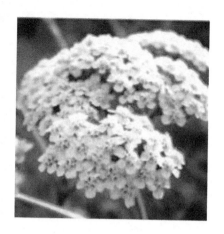

Yarrow plant (Achillea millefolium): is a perennial weed that comes from the aster family. It grows in yards, along roadsides, and in other disturbed places all over the United States. Interesting fact: the science name "Achillea" comes from Homer's epic poem "The Iliad." A hero named Achilles in that epic poem used yarrow to stop the wounds of his men during the Trojan War. There are chemicals in yarrow called alkaloids that can stop bleeding very quickly. Crush its leaves or flowers and put them on cuts and wounds. It can also help with digestion and nervousness, and it can reduce inflammation and ease pain. People often drink yarrow tea to get rid of colds and fevers. But be careful: yarrow is often mistaken for the very poisonous hemlock, so you need to be very sure that you are identifying the right plant. If you can safely identify it, you will be rewarded with a plant that is good for you and can be eaten or used as medicine.

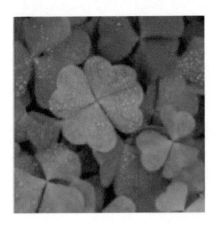

Clover (Trifolium spp.): You can easily spot both red and white clover in cooler, grassier parts of North America. These plants belong to the bean family. They are high in protein and help reduce inflammation. You can make tea out of the flowers or eat them raw in salads. They are full of vitamins and minerals. Clover is used by many women to treat menopause hot flashes and to get pregnant. Native Americans ate clover plants whole, even the roots, both raw and cooked.

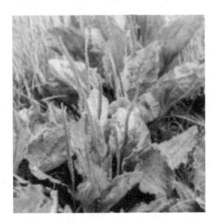

Plantain: If you want to see wild plantain, you can find it in backyards, along roadsides, and in cracks in city sidewalks. This plant can grow in rough spots where other plants can't. Also, it grows well most of the year in most areas, and its seeds can live for up to 40 years! It is possible to crush plantain leaves and use them as a bandage for cuts, rashes, poison ivy, snakebites, and nettle stings. They stop mosquito bites from hurting right away! There are three kinds that grow in large numbers in the US. All of them are good sources of iron, calcium, and magnesium, and are high in vitamins A, C, and K. You can eat young, tender plantain leaves raw, and older leaves are great added to soups and stews. You can also use them like kale or spinach, or bake them into plantain chips. This plant can kill bacteria and reduce inflammation. It is used to treat intestinal problems and improve health in general.

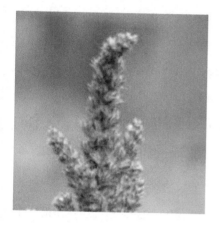

Amaranth: Another name for amaranth is pigweed. There are many types of amaranth that grow wild in the United States, and most of us can easily pick them. The greens are full of calcium, magnesium, vitamins A and C, and potassium. They can be cooked and used in a lot of different recipes. The seeds of amaranth can also be ground into flour that can be used in baking. Additionally, it feels great and is very healthy. Because of these things, you should learn how to recognize it and start gathering it!

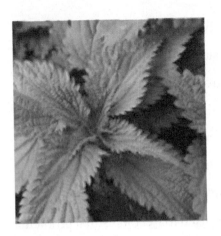

Nettle (Urtica dioica): The stinging leaves of this superfood make it hard to harvest. Be careful to cover any skin that is exposed, or you will feel the burning feeling of formic acid. But when you simmer or sauté it, the bitterness goes away, leaving you with one of the best wild greens around! This plant can be used like any other edible green. Pick only the tender tips and young plants that are less than two feet tall for the best taste. This weed that grows wild is good for reducing inflammation, killing bacteria, and tightening the skin. It's simple to find and wonderful.

If you look around, you can find hundreds of other useful plants. Some of my favorite plants are Echinacea, lobelia, berries, mullein, comfrey, wood sorrel, chickweed, sumac, and goldenrod. Fungi, like mushrooms, can also be used to find food, but you have to be very careful and good at identifying them because some species are very deadly and look a lot like edible ones. Because mushrooms can kill you quickly, we don't think that amateurs should collect them.

How To Safely Go Foraging

Foraging means going outside and picking plants, nuts, seeds, fungi, and veggies that you can eat. You can do this all year long, and it's a great way to spend time in nature. But you need to be careful to pick things that are safe to eat and in a way that doesn't harm the environment. Things you should know about wild plants before you start to forage are that some are dangerous and even deadly.

Sure to forage

Throughout the year, you can gather a wide range of wild foods. To get the most out of what the hedgerows have to give, use different parts of the same plants for different things. For example, elderberries are in season from late summer to fall and are often used to make jams and syrups. In the spring, elderflowers can be used to make drinks. You can still get blackberries and walnuts in late fall and early winter. You can find dandelion and burdock in the wild from spring to fall. The leaves can be used in salads, and the roots can be added to soups.

In the fall, there are also lots of wild mushrooms. But it's easy to get them mixed up, and some of them are very deadly. If you want to gather mushrooms from the wild, you should make sure you know what kind you are getting.

If you aren't sure what kind of mushrooms you are eating, you should never eat them.

Hemlock and hemlock water dropwort, which grows near water, are both carrot-like plants that look a lot like wild celery or turnip. Both, though, are toxic and could kill you.

Before you pick something, you should always be sure you know what it is. Leave it alone if you're not sure. When you go foraging, it's helpful to have a guidebook or an expert guide with you to help you figure out what is safe to eat and what could be harmful.

All over the UK, you can join a lot of organized foraging walks and foraging groups. Most of the time, foraging experts run these groups and can help you figure out how to identify and safely eat wild foods you've found.

People often gather plants and herbs from the wild, but that doesn't mean they are safe for everyone.

Some plants should not be eaten by people who are pregnant or who already have certain health problems. If you want to be safe, talk to a doctor or nurse before eating any foraged foods.

Also, know that just because some parts of a plant can be eaten doesn't mean all of them can be eaten. To get rid of poisons, some plants may need to be cooked. For example, elderberries need to be cooked to get rid of the poisons that are in them before they can be eaten. You should never eat the elder plant's leaves, bark, or roots.

Tips for safe foraging

- Always be sure of the plants you're collecting, because some of them are deadly
- Make sure to wash your harvest well, no matter where it came from
- If you want to eat wild food in a warm dish, like soup, cooking it until it's steaming hot will lower the risk of foodborne germs being present.
- Do not leave kids alone to pick or eat wild food.

- Don't pick any plant or fruit that looks like it's been hurt, like if it's bruised or moldy.

- Don't pick plants and berries that grow on or near old factories, busy roads, or areas where oil or ash can be seen on the ground.

- Don't pick plants that are close to built land or busy roads where pesticides may have been used.

- Do not pick from low-lying plants that may have been messed up by animals or from the ground.

- If you've never eaten a foraged food before, start by eating a small amount to make sure you don't have a bad response.

- Set a piece of the foraged food aside so that you can identify it if you eat it and get sick.

- Remember that when you go digging, you should only take what you need so that the plant can grow more.

It is against the Wildlife and Countryside Act 1981 (Opens in a new window) and the Wildlife (Northern Ireland) Order 1985 (Opens in a new window) to pull up any wild plant without the owner or person living on the land's consent. It is also against the law to pick, uproot, gather seeds from, or sell any species that is very rare or easily hurt.

Chapter 9

How To Be An Environmentally Sustainable Herbalist

As plant professionals, it is our duty to think about how our actions affect plant populations in order to make sure that future generations can use herbs as food and health aids. By doing these things, you can help protect our valuable plants and practice herbalism in a way that doesn't harm the earth.

Four Ways To Be An Herbalist Who Cares About the Environment

1. Herbs for Wildcraft

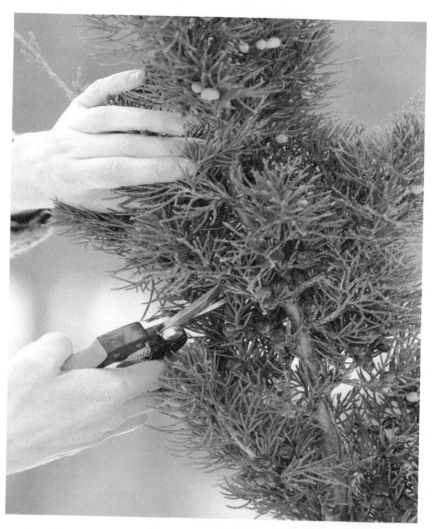

Wildcrafting, which is also called "foraging," is the act of gathering plants, mushrooms, and flowers from the wild. If you do it carefully and with plants that can keep giving you herbs, this can be a lasting way to get them because you are just using what nature has given you with no help from people.

Wildcrafting is a way for an environmentally friendly herbalist to reduce their impact on the environment by not having to ship herbs from far away.

It also helps them connect more deeply with the plants they gather and the land they live on. When it comes to making herbal medicines and adding herbs to food, the plants that grow nearby can be our best source. The plants that grow nearby are often in large amounts and can be found cheaply with some care and experience.

Although we can easily order a lot of different plants and have them sent right to our door, we might choose a more well-known species for our herbal needs when there is probably a similar plant in our own garden or in the area around us. Before you choose which herbs to use, look at what you can find in the nearby fields and woods and see if that plant can meet your needs and if its population can support harvesting.

It is important to learn about wildcrafting before you go on your first trip: it is very important to be able to identify the plants correctly, understand their environment and what they need, and follow good wildcrafting ethics and practical concerns.

2. Herbs from around the house

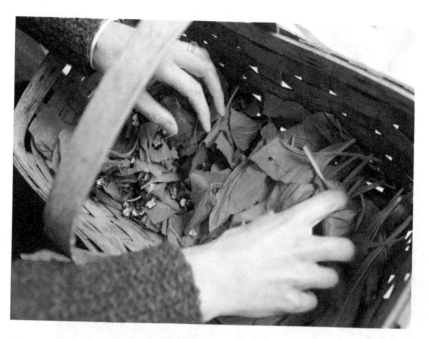

If you can't get flowers from the wild, you might need to buy them from a reliable source. Surprisingly, a lot of bulk herbs don't come from plants grown in the United States. It's possible that the greens you buy online are certified organic, but they could also be from Egypt, Croatia, or other places. Not only does buying herbs from thousands of miles away leave a big impact on the environment because of the journey, but it also means that the herb has had more time to go from being picked to being delivered, so it won't be as fresh!

Many herbs sold online come from places other than the United States. However, that doesn't mean you can't find herbs locally that meet your needs. In the United States, there are a lot of herb farms. You might be shocked (and lucky!) to find one close to where you live.

3. Don't use too many essential oils.

198

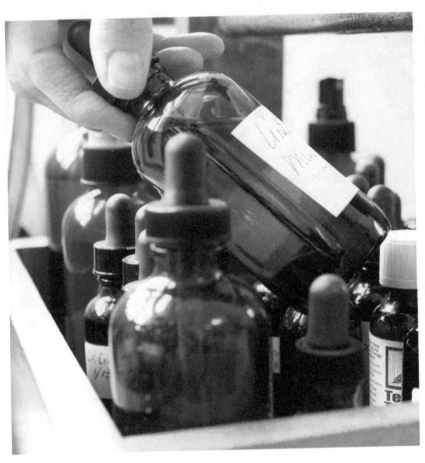

Essential oils are probably something you've used or at least heard a lot about if you're interested in natural health. You can use these volatile plant oils on your skin, in your hair, as a natural bug spray, in cleaning products, to help you stay healthy in the winter, to ease headaches, to heal wounds and scars, and they may even help people with Alzheimer's and dementia live better lives.

Essential oils can be used in many ways and offer many benefits when they are part of a balanced lifestyle. Along with these many benefits, there are some things you should know about essential oils. One of the most important is the problem of sustainability.

How essential oils are made is something that isn't talked about as much. It may take a lot of plant stuff to make one drop of essential oil for some plants. AromaWeb (n.d.) says that it can take fifty roses to make one drop of rose essential oil. As you think about how much time, energy, and natural resources are used to grow, harvest, and handle just one drop of essential oil, keep these things in mind.

It's important to use essential oils sparingly and to think about whether we really need to use them or if there is a better, more environmentally friendly choice. Instead of putting orange essential oil in a cleaner, for example, you could use the rinds of a whole orange, which would normally go to waste.

Because of problems with sustainability, you should use even less of the following essential oils (or none at all):

- Rosewood (Taxocara rosea)
- It smells like agarwood (Aquilaria malaccensis).
- Frankincense coming from Somalia (Boswellia carterii)
- The Spikenard bird (Nardostachys jatamansi)

4. Think about what a real "need" is.

Being a good manager of the earth means using things in a smart way. Is this something I really need? That's the first thing you should ask yourself before you consume, buy, or gain something. Because herbs can help our bodies in so many ways, we might want to stock up on all the herbs and herbal goods we can find.

Instead of giving in to the urge to buy everything, even if it's something good for us, we should think about which herbs to buy in bulk and why.

This will help us live more simply and sustainably. It's easier to keep things simple and have less of an effect on environments if you use herbs that are easy to find and grow.

More often than not, sustainability is good for us as well as the world. As an environmentally sustainable herbalist, you should think about where the plants you use come from and how they are grown. This way, you can be sure that future generations will be able to continue this old practice.

Some of the most environmentally friendly ways to practice herbalism are to get herbs from nearby farms whenever possible, be aware when using herbs and essential oils, and gather our own herbs from the area whenever possible.

Herbal Seed Suppliers and Nurseries: Ethical Sources for Medicinal Seeds & Plants

From our own fields and backyards, we can get the freshest medicine in the world. When we grow our own herbal medicine cabinet, we have a very close connection with the quality and honesty of the herbs. Because of this, it is very important to start with healthy seeds and plants that have been grown naturally!

You might be thinking what makes a healthy source of seeds for medicines. These words are used to talk about different kinds of seeds and plants, and they all have something to do with herbs.

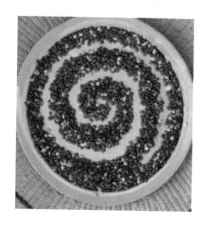

Passionflower seeds (Passiflora incarnata) that have just been cleaned.

Heirloom seeds come from old stock; their ancestors are usually types that were popular before World War II and have been passed down from generation to generation. Heirlooms are usually local types that have had certain traits picked out by hand over the years. Heirloom seeds are open-pollinated, and from season to season, their traits tend to stay the same (true to seed). In the world of vegetables, heirloom varieties are more popular than in herbal medicines and food. A lot of herbs have been grown for a very long time, with seeds being passed down from generation to generation. However, there aren't many named regional varieties or heirloom kinds of herbs.

Open-fertilized seeds are pollinated by bugs, birds, the wind, and other natural things, without any help from people. Most of the time, these seeds are easy to save and grow exactly as they should. Free-range plants are used to make almost all herbal seeds that are sold.

Hybrid seeds are made by crossing-pollinating two species or two types of the same species to get the traits that people want. Many plant groups (genera) naturally hybridize. For thousands of years, people have been crossing plants to get traits they want. Do not mix up mixed seeds with GMO seeds! They're not the same at all.

Yes, there are some great crosses out there. Just remember that they are not as true to seed from year to year as open-pollinated seeds. There is no way to know what traits the plants you save from will have when they grow up, but it's likely that they won't have the traits of their parent plant. Most of the time, mixed herbs don't come in seeds, but sometimes they do come in pots.

Cultivars, which are short for "cultivated varieties," are made when two plants are crossed, plants are picked, or plants change naturally. To stay true to type, cultivars usually need to be spread without pollination, such as by split or cuttings. Because of this, it's better to buy starts (small potted plants that have been split) of peppermint or chocolate mint types than to grow them from seeds, since the offspring won't usually have the same traits as the parent plant. If you grow it from a seed, you'll get a mint mutt!

GMO (genetically modified) plants have had their genes changed in a lab to make them have certain traits. This can be done by gene-splicing or other methods. While it's still not clear what the long-term effects of GMOs will be, some worries include the loss of genetic variety (because GMOs can cross-pollinate with other plants) and effects on ecology and animal health, such as in humans, insects, and other animals.

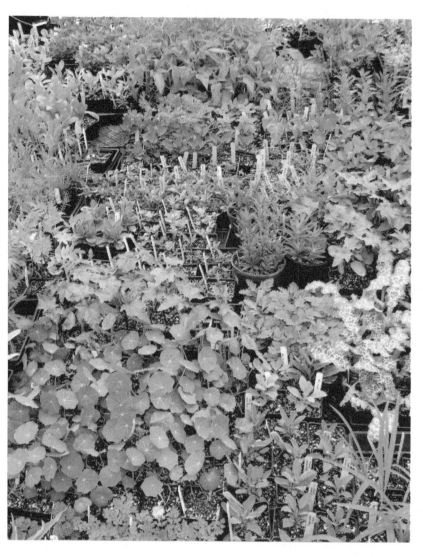

Chestnut Herb Nursery: Treating seeds in a certain way makes them grow into special plants.

You probably don't need me to go on and on about how important it is to protect seed sovereignty or how dangerous it is for mega-corporations to take control of our seeds by patenting them, changing them, and deciding how they are distributed.

That being said, I will say that in this age of big agriculture, it is important to give our money to seed savers who are ethical, organic, and sustainable.

A list of seed and herb businesses that mostly use organic methods or get their plants from organic farms (even if they're not "certified organic"). Still, you should check out each source on your own; some seed sellers sell both conventionally grown and organic seeds. Some are well-known plant businesses that have been around for a long time, while others are smaller and newer to growing scenes across the country.

Many of these companies ship goods all over the world, but if you'd rather keep things local, you should look for suppliers in your area. You'll notice that we've also made a separate list of small-scale and regional US suppliers. Also, keep in mind that this is not a complete list.

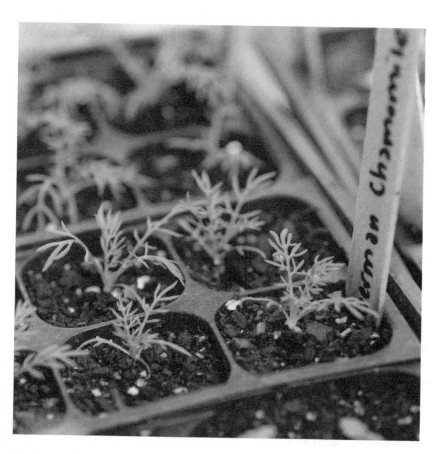

German chamomile (Matricaria recutita) began in a window that faced south.

Companies that sell and grow herbal seeds in the United States

Fedco Plants

A seed and garden supply company in Maine that is run by its members. Offers a large selection of local plants, herbs used for medicine and cooking, and shrubs and trees that can be eaten. It focuses on cold-hardy types. It also has a great guide on how to plant herbs seeds.

Johnny's Picked Seeds

A lot of seeds and plants to choose from, including some that are healthy. A great place to get all the supplies you need for your farm, like yard tools, soil amendments, and more.

Good Farms in Peaceful Valley

A lot of organic seeds, plants, and soil improvers, as well as a wide range of garden tools and supplies for starting seeds and growing plants.

The Prairie Moon Nursery

My favorite place to learn about plants that are native to the eastern and central United States. The prices are very low, the plants are grown organically (but not certified), and the business is run by a cooperative.

Seeds for Southern Exposure

Heirloom kinds, with a focus on types that do well in the southeast and mid-Atlantic parts of the US.

Seeds Only for Medical Use

This Oregon-based company, which used to be called Horizon Herbs, has the biggest selection of medicinal herb seeds and plants that are grown organically. For over twenty years, it's been one of my go-tos.

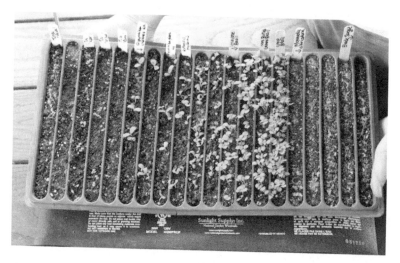

An electric heat mat is warming up a row tray with a lot of seedlings that will be poked out and moved to bigger cells before they are planted outside.

Suppliers in the United States that are small and local

Businesses run by Black, Indigenous, and People of Color (BIPOC) people are written in purple.

Group of Native Seed Keepers

The goal of selling medicinal and edible herb, flower, and vegetable seeds is to bring back the spiritual connections between Native Americans and plants.

The Black Locust Gardens

The medicinal herb farm and nursery is in Dexter, MI, and it sells standard medicinal herb starts and a few medicinal shrubs all year long. You can buy plants online, but you have to pick them up in person. Getting organic certification in the spring of 2019.

Plants to go with

Outside of Athens, Ohio, there is a herb garden. They have over 200 different kinds of seeds and a lot of different kinds of herb plants, most of which they grow themselves in ways that are good for the climate.

Nursery of Crimson Sage Medical Plants

A wide range of rare and threatened live medicinal plants, including plants used in Chinese and Ayurvedic medicine and many hard-to-find European and Native American herbs. Verified to be organic. A small business in northwest California that is run by a woman.

Seeds for Earthbeat

A seed company in Vermont that focuses on medicinal herbs and plants that draw native pollinators. Earthbeat Seeds works with small-scale growers all over the country who grow their crops in an ethical way and use only recycled, unbleached, and compostable packages.

Seeds of Eloheh

Herb, flower, and veggie seeds that are grown organically, don't contain GMOs, are open-pollinated, and come straight from the farm. The office is in Oregon at the Eloheh Indigenous Center for Earth Justice.

Plants that Friends of the Trees grows

Medicinal herb seeds that were found in the wild or grown in the Pacific Northwest using organic ways.

Herbs and foods from the garden

The business is run by a cooperative and sells a wide range of ecologically grown, open-pollinated medicinal seeds, some of which are certified organic. Set up in Virginia.

The Exchange for Growers

It does not sell seeds but does sell rare vegetable plants that are not genetically modified. Set up in Virginia.

The Good Seed Company.

Heirloom and open-pollinated non-GMO seeds that are adapted to the area. These seeds include medicinal herbs, veggies, and flowers that were chosen for their value in homesteading and permaculture. It is based in Whitefish, Montana.

The Wild Mountain Herbs by Harding

Gives American Ginseng (Panax quinquefolius) seeds and rootlets for growing. With roots in Maryland.

Early Summer Farm's Herb Farm

A certified organic nursery in Warwick, NY that grows medicinal and native plants. They are only open on certain times during the growing season.

Apple Valley Seed Co.

Herb, flower, and veggie seeds that are certified organic, heirloom, and open-pollinated. Located in New York.

The Native Seed Initiative

A place to get non-GMO, historically important, wild and garden-grown seeds from Asia, Africa, Europe, Central and South America, and North America.

Garden of Medicine

This is a medicinal plant nursery in Portland, OR, that has a lot of traditional and local herbs.

Organics that are tanned

We have the best non-hybrid, healthy organic seeds to help you grow great food. You should sell some herbs that can be used for both food and medicine. There is also a range of flower and veggie seeds. A small range of garden items.

Mountain Views

This is Joe Hollis's botanical yard. He teaches here at the Chestnut School of Herbal Medicine on the side. You can order seeds and bare root plants by mail. They focus on Appalachian and Chinese therapeutic herbs. Mountain Gardens may be harder to get seeds from than other places, but the huge range and high quality are well worth the extra work. It is based in North Carolina.

Look for Native Seeds

A nonprofit seed protection group based in Tucson, Arizona. Their goal is to protect and spread the variety of drought-tolerant plants (including herbs) that grow in the Southwest to help farming remain sustainable and ensure food security. Through the Native American Seed Request

Program, Native Seeds Search tries to make sure that Native Americans can still get these traditional seeds.

Dope by Nature

Do you want a cool garden? This is a small-scale place to get CBD seeds and plant seeds used for medicine.

Plants from Panaea

This is a botanical refuge and biodynamic herb nursery in North Carolina. You can ship plant starts across the country or pick them up in person.

The Herb Garden Thyme Co.

Organically grown, non-GMO flower seeds and live plants for cooking and medicine. With roots in Oregon.

Seeds of true love

Rare, open-pollinated flower, herb, and vegetable seeds that are traditionally significant are for sale. All of their farms are dedicated to seed sovereignty and farming that doesn't harm the environment. Set up in Philadelphia, PA.

Nursery of Useful Plants

Chuck Marsh started the garden based on permaculture. Marsh is a famous teacher and permaculturist who has since left this world. They focus on helpful, phytonutritional medicine and food plants that do well in the southern Appalachians and nearby bioregions.

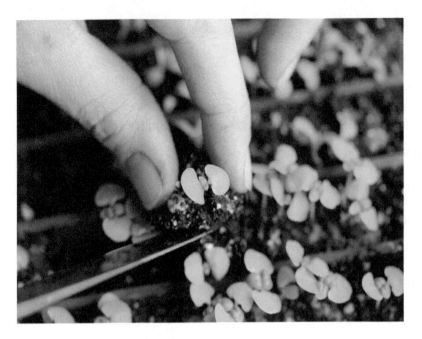

Making holes in a basil bud so that it can be moved to a tray with bigger cells.

Nurseries and companies that sell herbal seeds in Canada

Herbs that Sing

An AB family business sells a range of non-GMO, open-pollinated medicinal herb seeds, as well as veggie, flower, and grain seeds.

Seeds for Raven Songs

A small seed company on Vancouver Island, BC, grows medicinal plants that are grown organically. They also sell a variety of culinary herbs, flowers, vegetables, and garlic.

The Richters

This Canadian nursery has a huge range of herb seeds and plants, some of which are rare or hard to find. It sells uncommon plants. With roots in Toronto.

Seeds from Salt Spring

Heirloom seeds for veggies, grains, herbs for cooking and medicine, and plants that attract pollinators.

Chapter 10
Guide to Herbalist Terminology

It might be a little overwhelming to keep track of herbal words, whether you are an expert herbalist or just a passionate about herbs. Here's an A-Z list of essential herbalist phrases to know while you enjoy your cup of herbal tea or take in your newly planted herb garden. It's always good to have a quick reference sheet on hand!

Adaptogens: Herbs that help the body better adjust to stress are known as adaptogens. Adaptogens support wellbeing, health, and balance. They generally aid in the restoration of normal organ and system functioning.

Adjuvant: These herbs improve how well the body reacts to a treatment. It supports the activity of other substances in a formula that balance energetic properties, promote absorption, or accelerate the whole reaction.

Allopathy: Another word for standard, contemporary Western medicine is allopathic medicine. Doctors and other medical professionals treat symptoms using traditional drugs within an evidence-based approach.

Alterative: these substances aid the body's gradual return to its typical state of health, energy, and function. Not all alteratives are adaptogens, but all adaptogens are alteratives.

Analgesic: A drug that reduces pain is called an analgesic.

Anodyne: Anodyne is another word for a painkilling substance. It functions by lessening the perception of or response from the neurological system.

Anthelmintic: Vermifuge is another word for anthelmintic, and these herbs aid in the removal of worms from the digestive tract.

Antiemetics: Herbs known as "antiemetics" are used to lessen nausea and either stop or stop vomiting.

Aperient: The term "aperient" is generally employed to characterize a moderate laxative. Aperients are generally utilized to prepare the digestive environment and also promote appetite and digestion.

Astringent: Herbs classified as astringents tighten and strengthen tissues. Herbs that are astringent tighten and tone the body. They control bodily secretions as well.

Apothecary: is a person who prepares and delivers medication or a location where it is done so.

Aromatherapy: is the use of plant materials (usually but not always essential oils) to enhance health and well-being. Plant extracts are used in aromatherapy for both therapeutic and aesthetic effects.

Ayurveda: is the result of conjugating the Sanskrit terms "ayus," which means "life," and "veda," which means "science." Ayurveda is a collection of teachings that relate to an age-old Indian medical system that promotes vigorous health via the use of foods, herbs, yoga breathing, and lifestyle choices.

Balsamic: Herb that reduces and calms inflammation is balsamic.

Carminative: The volatile oils of carminative herbs help to soothe the stomach and stimulate the digestive tract. Plants that are carminative aid in avoiding gas.

Compress: A compress is a topical treatment used to reduce pain or inflammation and soften tissue. A cloth soaked in a herbal liquid preparation, such as a decoction or tea, is used to make it. After wringing it dry, the cloth is applied externally to the skin or body.

Decoction: Simmering or boiling plant components results in a concentrated water extraction. The denser portions of the plant, such as the bark, roots, berries, mushrooms, and seeds, are usually treated with it. Compared to an infusion, a decoction is more concentrated.

Demulcent: A mucilaginous plant that covers mucous membranes with a calming coating. When discussing internal use, the word demulcent is used. A common remedy for sore throats is slippery elm, which is a demulcent.

Depurative: These herbs are thought to have cleansing or purifying properties.

Diuretic: Promotes increased urine production and excretion.

Emetics: These are the vomiting-inducing herbs.

Emollient: Skin-protecting, skin-softening, skin-soothing substances. Unlike a demulcent, which is intended for internal use, the phrase refers to external use.

Emmenagogue: By acting on the liver, these medicines serve to restore hormone levels and encourage and control menstrual flow.

Essential oil: They're not really oils, despite their name. Distillation is the process used to create high-quality essential oils. They can be further classified as hydrocarbons or oxygenated compounds based on their chemical makeup. The aroma of essential oils is strong.

Expectorant: These herbs help the body clear the respiratory system of extra mucus.

Glyceract: Vegetable glycerine is used in place of alcohol to make this tincture. Although glyercine is chemically categorized as alcohol, it lacks the detrimental consequences of alcohol, such as drunkenness. Glyceracts are commonly prescribed for animals, kids, and people who are sensitive to alcohol.

Herbal medicine: Using medicinal plants to cure illnesses and promote overall health and well-being, herbal medicine has its roots in ancient cultures.

Herbalism: The science and practice of employing plants to nourish the body, mind, and spirit in order to promote healing and overall well-being is known as herbalism. Additionally, ceremonial folklore and cultural symbolism are included in herbalism. Using plant extracts or whole plants in meals, herbal tea, powered herbs, smudges, liquid extracts, skin treatments, and incense are examples of this practice.

Homeopathy: The "like cures like" notion is the basis of this medical approach. According to the American Botanical Council (2016), it is the process of preparing diluted plant, mineral, or animal ingredients that are "matched to specific symptom pattern profiles of illness to stimulate the body's natural healing process."

Hepatic: They improve the liver's strength and tone while also boosting bile flow.

Hypnotics: Herbal remedies that promote restful sleep. They don't put people in a hypnotic state.

Infusion: An infusion is a medicinal treatment or extract that is prepared by immersing plant material in a liquid, usually water. For flowers and leaves that have volatile oils, easily extracted vitamins, and enzymes that may be dissolved in hot water, infusions are advised.

Infusion Oil: Oil that has had the properties of a herb infused into it over a period of time, ranging from hours to weeks, with the possibility of applying heat.

Liniment: A liquid lotion applied topically to ease discomfort, formulated with oils.

Macerating: The procedure of macerating a herb involves slicing or grinding it, putting it in a jar, and then covering it with a solvent (alcohol and water). After letting this combination sit for a while, it is strained out. The plant's extracted active ingredients are found in the tincture, which is the remaining liquid.

Materia Medica: The corpus of knowledge gathered concerning materials with medicinal characteristics is referred to as materia medica. This would be the collective knowledge of herbs and plant materials for herbalists.

Mucilage: is a polysaccharide material that gives some plants their gelatinous consistency when removed.

Nervine: These herbs have a variety of activities and are good for the nervous system. While some of them tone and strengthen, others stimulate or relax.

Pharmacognosy: is the study of pharmaceuticals derived from plants or animals. A definition provided by the American Society of Pharmacognosy is: "the study of the physical, chemical, biochemical, and biological properties of drugs, drug substances, or potential drugs or drug substances of natural origin as well as the search for new drugs from natural sources."

Poultice: Applying a moist, soft mass of plant material topically to a wound is known as a poultice. Herbs that have been poulticed are often secured in place with a cloth, bandage, leaf, or other appropriate object.

Rubefacient: These agents dilate capillaries close to the skin's surface when administered topically, causing mild local irritation. Deeper interior pain is reduced as a result of increased circulation and the release of congestion or inflammation.

Sedative: These herbs ease tension and anxiety by soothing the nervous system. Additionally, they support body parts that are impacted by neurological issues.

Solar Infusion: Plant materials soaked in oil are usually used to make solar infusion. After sealing the jar, it is placed in the sun to allow the heat from the sun to release the phytochemical into the oil.

Salve: A semi-solid herbal concoction with fat content that is typically applied externally. Generally speaking, the ingredients consist of softened beeswax and an oil, such as extra virgin olive oil flavored with herbs.

Tincture: A tincture is a plant extract prepared by soaking plants in glycerine, vinegar, or alcohol for two to six weeks in a dark location. The plant material is filtered out of this liquid, and the herbal tincture is then applied topically.

Tonics: Herbs that energise, invigorate, and fortify the body are known as tonics.

Vulnerary: These herbs help the body heal cuts and wounds when applied topically.

Made in the USA
Las Vegas, NV
21 March 2024

87521837R10125